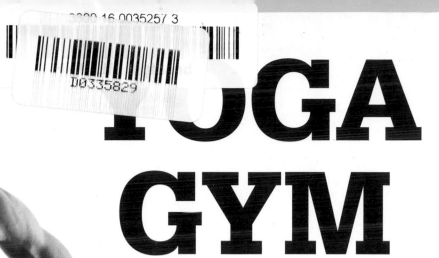

# YOGA GYM

The revolutionary 28 day plan for strength, flexibility and fat loss

Nicola Jane Hobbs

## B L O O M S B U R Y

LONDON · NEW DELHI · NEW YORK · SYDNEY

D0335829

**NOTE:** No responsibility for loss caused to any individual or organization acting on or refraining from action as a result of the material in this publication can be accepted by Bloomsbury or the author.

**Bloomsbury Sport**

**An imprint of Bloomsbury Publishing Plc**

| 50 Bedford Square | 1385 Broadway |
|---|---|
| London | New York |
| WC1B 3DP | NY 10018 |
| UK | USA |

www.bloomsbury.com

BLOOMSBURY and the Diana logo are trademarks of Bloomsbury Publishing Plc

First published 2016

© Nicola Jane Hobbs, 2016

Nicola Jane Hobbs has asserted her right under the Copyright, Designs and Patents Act, 1988, to be identified as Author of this work.

All rights reserved. No part of this publication may be reproduced or transmitted in any form or by any means, electronic or mechanical, including photocopying, recording, or any information storage or retrieval system, without prior permission in writing from the publishers.

British Library Cataloguing-in-Publication Data

A catalogue record for this book is available from the British Library.

Library of Congress Cataloguing-in-Publication data has been applied for.

ISBN: Print: 9781472912886

ePDF: 9781472912909

ePub: 9781472912893

10 9 8 7 6 5 4 3

Bloomsbury Publishing Plc makes every effort to ensure that the papers used in the manufacture of our books are natural, recyclable products made from wood grown in well-managed forests. Our manufacturing processes conform to the environmental regulations of the country of origin.

...........................................................................................................................................

**ACKNOWLEDGEMENTS:** Cover photograph © Geoff Whitaker

Inside photographs © Eddie Macdonald

Hair and make-up artist: Alice Hollinghum

Models: Nicola Jane Hobbs and Edd Lawrence

Design: Nicola Liddiard, Nimbus Design

Printed and bound in China by RRD Asia Printing Solutions Limited

To find out more about our authors and books visit www.bloomsbury.com. Here you will find extracts, author interviews, details of forthcoming events and the option to sign up for our newsletters.

# Contents

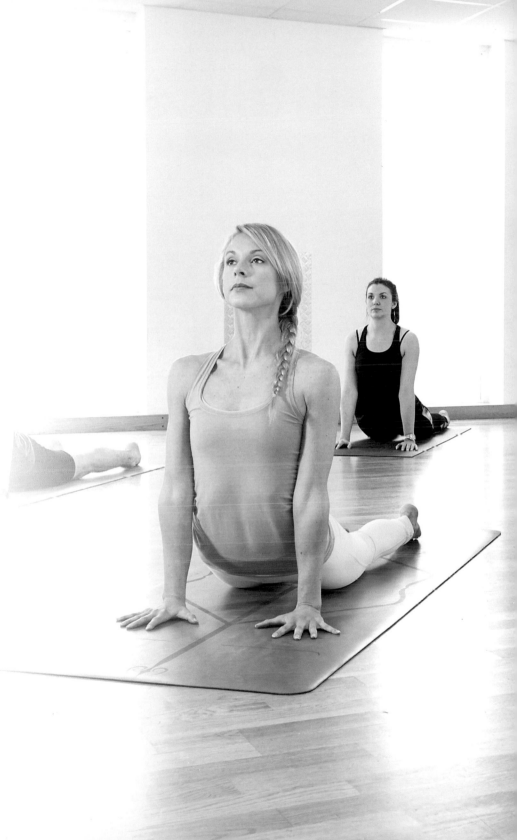

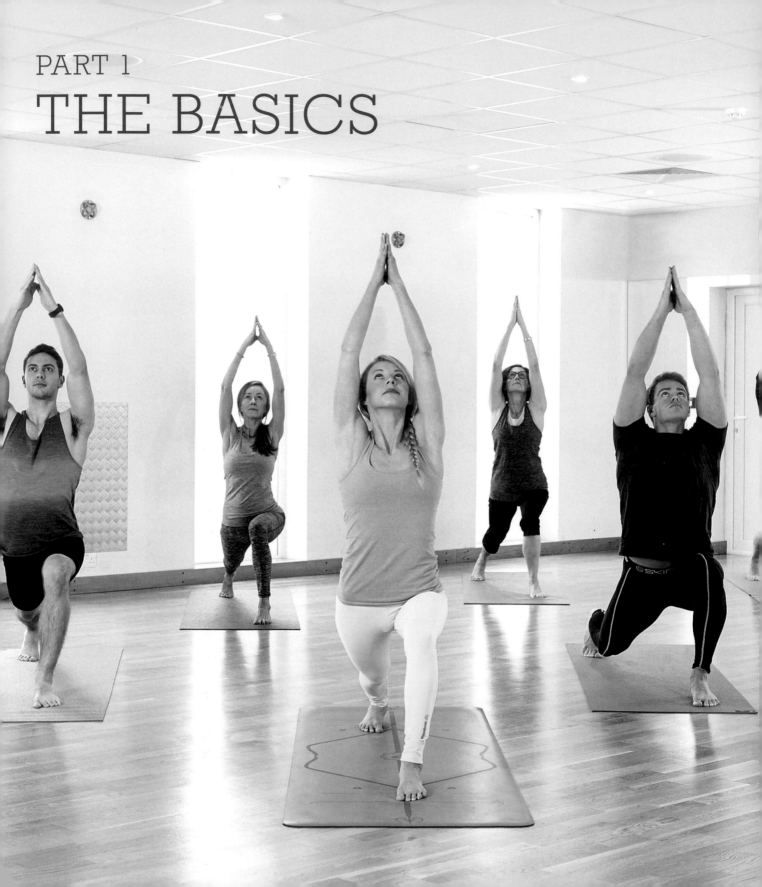

PART 1
# THE BASICS

# Introduction

**I want you to understand that you are the expert of your own body.**

Intuitively, you know how to move it, train it and nourish it. The health and fitness world has become so cluttered with overcomplicated workout machines, the latest gadgets and gizmos and miracle potions in a bottle that you have forgotten the innate power of your body. Nutrition companies battle it out over the best diet. Coaches argue over the optimal amount of weight to lift or distance to run. Yogis deliberate over the finest and truest form of yoga. All this confusion paralyses us in a state of inaction.

I have created Yoga Gym so you can get healthier, stronger and leaner with peace of mind  No more complicated equipment. No more crowded gyms. No more confusion. We have become so advanced in fitness that we have forgotten the basics – how to breathe, stand, move, and how to build our body *using* our body.

This book offers a simplicity that the health and fitness world desperately needs. This simplicity means that people of all ages, genders, occupations and athletic ability can follow the Yoga Gym plan. Each pose and exercise in this book has been refined through my work with professional athletes, by teaching corporate office workers and full-time parents, and by coaching children of all ages. I've developed the plan using yoga in weight-loss groups, helping individuals through eating disorders and depression and supporting war veterans with post-traumatic stress disorder, and have used the power of yoga to inspire individuals, families and communities to thrive.

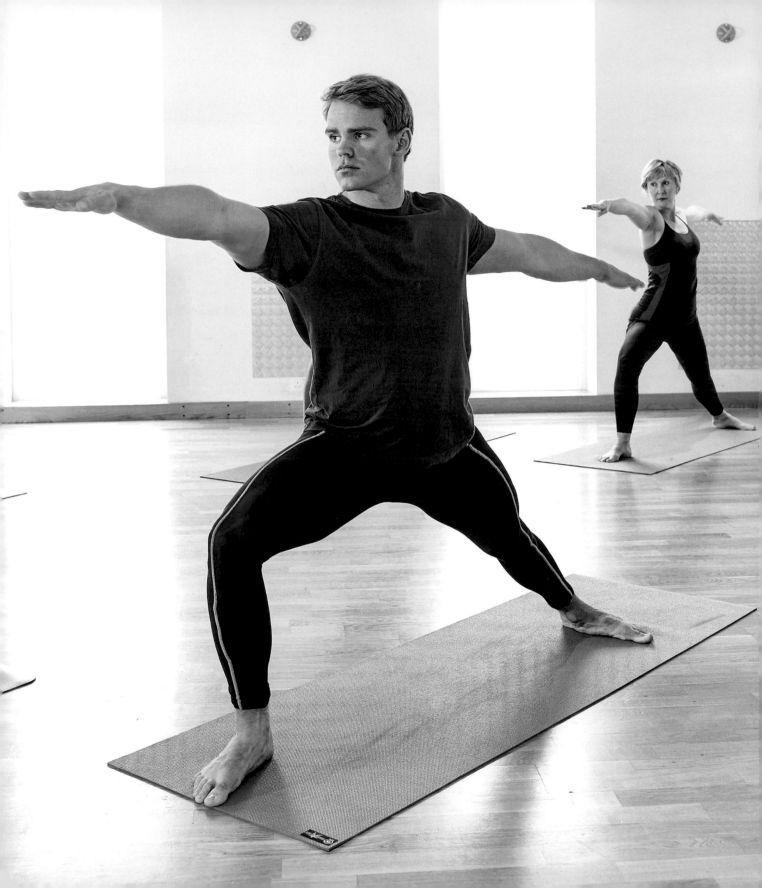

# What is Yoga Gym?

Yoga Gym is a revolutionary approach to fitness that unites the ancient science of yoga with modern strength and conditioning principles. It provides you with over 150 equipment-free, do-anywhere poses and exercises as well as a 28-day life-enhancing plan to get you strong and flexible from head to toe.

The poses and exercises in this book are all based around traditional yoga poses known as 'asanas'. These come from various systems of yoga including:

**ASHTANGA** PHYSICALLY DEMANDING POSES PERFORMED IN A SET SEQUENCE

**IYENGAR** CHALLENGING POSES WITH A FOCUS ON CORRECT ALIGNMENT

**VINYASA FLOW** LIVELY AND FAST-PACED BREATH-SYNCHRONISED MOVEMENT

**YIN** PASSIVE POSES HELD FOR LONGER PERIODS TO TARGET THE CONNECTIVE TISSUES AND ENCOURAGE RELAXATION

In Sanskrit, the traditional Indo-Aryan language of yoga, these asanas have names such as 'Adho Mukha Svanasa' and 'Salamba Sarvangasana'. Although these terms are beautiful, they can be intimidating and alienating if you have never done yoga before or aren't interested in its history. For this reason, I have used modern, easy-to-understand pose names and movement cues in this book to authentically evolve yoga and make it more accessible to 21st century living.

As yoga means to 'yolk' or 'unite' in Sanskrit, I have united traditional poses with bodyweight training exercises known as calisthenics. Calisthenics has a long history dating back to the ancient Greeks (the word 'calisthenics' comes from the Greek 'kalli' meaning 'beautiful' and 'sthenos' meaning 'strength'). It includes exercises such as push-ups, pull-ups and squats, which I have drawn upon to create yogacises – yoga-based bodyweight exercises used to achieve bodily fitness and grace of movement.

# Why did I create it?

I'm not a classical yogi. I eat meat. I wear make-up. I probably don't meditate enough. And I definitely haven't reached spiritual enlightenment. I am just a girl journeying through life trying to share the joys of health, strength and freedom.

As a yoga teacher, I was tired of seeing men avoiding yoga classes in case they were the only ones who couldn't touch their toes. As a champion weightlifter, I was fed up with seeing women afraid to train for strength for fear of becoming bulky. And as a performance and lifestyle coach, I was frustrated by seeing people shy away from leading a healthy life because they were too ashamed of their body to exercise in public, they didn't know what to eat or how to move, or they simply didn't believe they were worthy of health and happiness.

So the reason for creating Yoga Gym is simple: to provide you with the tools to understand and master your body so you can become a stronger, healthier and more confident you.

This can be broken down into four main aims:

**1 To improve the fitness and function of the body**
If you walk into a standard commercial gym it is highly likely you will find lines of men and women gliding up and down on **elliptical trainers** (also known as cross-trainers). Sure, you might burn a few calories on these stationary machines but gliding is not a natural body motion. Yoga Gym gets you moving your body in the way it was designed to, so you condition it to perform better at everyday activities such as standing, bending and lifting. It builds fitness on all levels, including strength, power, flexibility and cardiovascular endurance to give you a better-functioning body that will last a lifetime.

**2 To improve body composition**
One of the main reasons we exercise is to look good. Sometimes we're too ashamed to admit that we would like to lose belly fat or tighten up our thighs for fear of being judged as vain. However, vanity can be a powerful motivator to work out. Embrace those feelings and notice how your body develops new lines and curves with a healthy definition and firmness as you improve your **body composition** by losing fat and building muscle.

### 3  To improve athletic performance

As a former national champion in Olympic weightlifting, I have experienced the benefits of yoga, when done correctly, in relation to sporting performance. Most athletes tend to be very driven, adrenaline-addicted folks with perfectionist personalities, so Yoga Gym is designed to develop peak performance by bringing the body back into equilibrium. By focusing on alignment and the subtle sensations of the body, you gain better body awareness, mobility and functional strength for your next training session, meaning you can become a more balanced athlete.

### 4  To improve mental well-being

As you gain physical strength, you will become stronger mentally, so you can persevere through challenges. As you increase the flexibility of your limbs, you will develop psychological flexibility so you can use the right emotional resources to create the kind of life you want. And as you lose fat to build a healthy body, you will be able to let go of any mental baggage that weighs you down. By giving yourself time each day to work out you are nourishing your body, mind and spirit, and cultivating health, happiness and well-being on all levels.

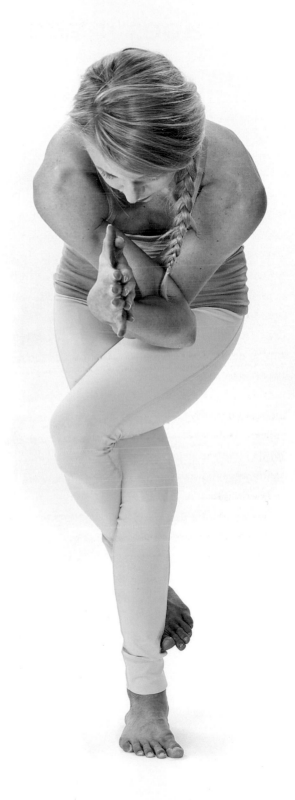

# How does it work?

There are over 150 yoga poses and yogacises in this book. The first thing to do is to explore them. Learn the alignment, the movement, which muscles to contract and which muscles to relax. Get to grips with your current strengths and weaknesses and which variation of the pose or yogacise gets you working just outside your comfort zone (use the strength and flexibility tests on p. 12 as a guide). There is no one to impress, so take the time to get to know your body and how to hold it, move it and use it optimally.

Once you are familiar with the poses and yogacises you can embark on the Yoga Gym plan. This lasts for 28 days and consists of five workouts a week, targeting different body parts and using varying intensities and training techniques. The plan has been designed, tested and refined to give you everything you need to increase your strength and flexibility; improve the metabolic, neurological and biomechanical function of your body; reduce stress levels; and give you a kick-start to get in the best shape possible. Although the plan has been designed to be completed in 28 days, don't worry if you need to spread out the workouts and it takes you a little longer.

Once you have completed the plan, either repeat it using more challenging variations of each pose and yogacise, or have a go at constructing your own workouts. If you are a confident yogi, calisthenics' fan or have experience in strength and conditioning exercises then you might want to jump right in and create your own training plan. With so many poses and yogacises, the combinations are infinite. Each pose and yogacise in Part 2 highlights the key areas of the body it strengthens and stretches, so use this in combination with the guidance notes in Part 3 on the benefits of different training techniques to develop a regime to suit your goals.

The Yoga Gym plan and exercises can replace most other fitness regimes: it can be used as a supplement to other types of training such as weightlifting, running or team sports, or you can pack this book in your bag for when you're going away and don't have access to a gym. Whether done in a living room, hotel room, garden, beach, office or athletics track, Yoga Gym works because you can use it any time and anywhere so there is no excuse not to become healthier, fitter and stronger.

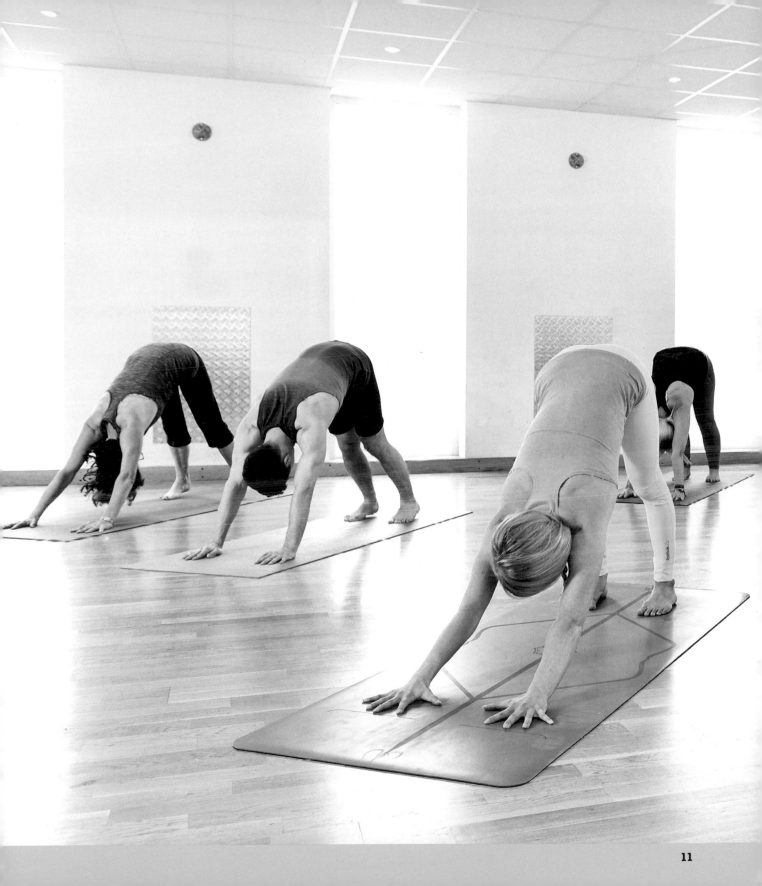

# Quick-start guide

I know you are keen to get started on your Yoga Gym journey so I've created the Simple, Strong and Stretchy Workout that you can do as you're reading through the rest of Part 1. If you can't wait to start the full plan then you can jump straight to Part 3 (see p. 197) and flick back to read about the Yoga Gym benefits, diet, and mindset tips when you have time. Just make sure you read over the key concepts on p. 47 and test your current strength and flexibility levels using the table below so you can choose the right level of pose and yogacise to suit your fitness.

# Strength & flexibility test

Some yoga poses and yogacises in the book come with different variations and progressions. You can test your strength and flexibility before you begin by performing the five fitness tests below. Hold the poses in the static strength tests for as long as you can. For the dynamic strength tests, do as many **repetitions** as you can with no rest until you can't do any more. You may find that your upper body is stronger than your lower body or vice versa, so look at the target area of each pose and yogacise in Part 2 and select the option best suited to your aims.

Use your results as a guide and listen to your body. An exercise is only as good as the posture in which you perform it, so always remember to do a less challenging version of the pose or yogacise if you need to.

Taking 'before' and 'after' photographs of yourself can help you to track your progress. You can use the hashtag #YogaGym to share your progress.

## YOGA POSE AND YOGACISE OPTIONS

| TYPE OF FITNESS | TEST POSE OR YOGACISE | VARIATION | STANDARD (MAIN IMAGE AND DESCRIPTION) | PROGRESSION |
|---|---|---|---|---|
| UPPER BODY STATIC STRENGTH | Plank (see p. 84) | <45 seconds | 45–60 seconds | >60 seconds |
| LOWER BODY STATIC STRENGTH | Chair (see p. 62) | <45 seconds | 45–60 seconds | >60 seconds |
| UPPER BODY DYNAMIC STRENGTH | Push-ups (see p. 122) | <10 | 10–16 | >20 |
| LOWER BODY DYNAMIC STRENGTH | Squats (see p. 135) | <12 | 12–20 | >20 |
| FULL BODY FLEXIBILITY | Forward Bend (see p. 65) | Fingertips above ankles | Fingertips between ankles and toes | Fingertips to floor |

# Simple, strong & stretchy workout

---

**1 ROUND**

Four Face Breathing (see p. 54)

---

**1 ROUND**

1 minute x Cat & Cow (see p. 111)

1 minute x Forward Bend Flow (see p. 114)

---

**1 ROUND**

5 breaths x Down Dog (see p. 80)

5 breaths x Plank (see p. 84)

5 breaths x Baby Cobra (yang) (see p. 101)

5 breaths x Up Dog (see p. 102)

5 breaths x Mountain (see p. 59)

5 breaths x Tree (see p. 76)

5 breaths x Chair (see p. 62)

5 breaths x Standing Forward Bend (see p. 65)

---

**3 ROUNDS**

12 x Classic Push-ups (see p. 122)

*Push off a wall or elevate hands on a surface if necessary.*

Rest @ 60 seconds

---

**3 ROUNDS**

12 x Squats (see p. 135)

Rest @ 60 seconds

---

**3 ROUNDS**

12 x Hinges (see p. 151)

Rest @ 60 seconds

---

**3 ROUNDS**

12 x Glute Bridges (see p. 147)

Rest @ 60 seconds

---

**1 ROUND**

20 breaths x Melting Heart (see p. 179)

20 breaths x Caterpillar (see p. 182)

20 breaths x Butterfly (yin) (see p. 167)

20 breaths x Sleeping Butterfly (see p. 167)

40 breaths x Corpse (see p. 193)

# Success stories

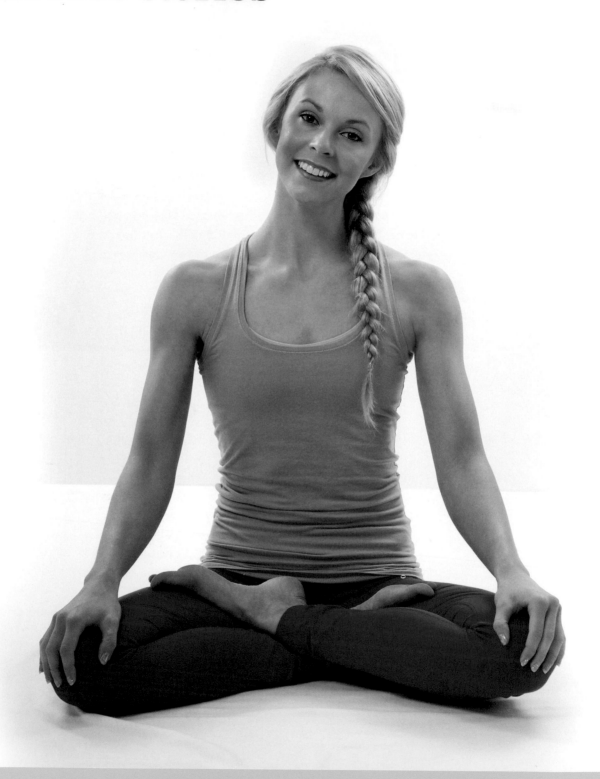

# My story

Yoga saved my life. I stumbled across it as a teenager in my local gym. I had been battling anorexia and depression for years and I was immediately drawn to the way yoga made me feel – strong, peaceful and free to explore who I was and who I wanted to be.

At this point, I'd been fighting an eating disorder since I was 15. I'd been in and out of various treatment centres and tried every therapy going. At 18, I hit rock bottom and had a near-death experience when I weighed just 25kg (55lb). My bones were riddled with osteoporosis. I'd gone deaf. I was depressed, drained and defeated. When I discovered yoga, my whole world changed. I regained weight and health, I went to Thailand to train as a yoga teacher, did a Master's degree in sport and exercise psychology, became English champion in Olympic weightlifting, and started writing *Yoga Gym* to challenge stereotypes, inspire hope and empower you to step outside of your comfort zone and be whatever and whoever you want to be.

Admittedly, sharing my story is pretty scary. After all, anorexia is messy. But sometimes you have to turn that mess into a message. *Yoga Gym* is my message. It is a message that you deserve to be the healthiest, fittest, strongest version of yourself. It is a message that being healthy is not about having the perfect body, the perfect diet, or the perfect exercise regime. Being healthy is not about becoming perfect; it is about becoming whole – uniting body, mind, heart and spirit to live life to the fullest.

Yoga transformed me from anorexic to athlete. It gave me a strong body that can run, jump and cartwheel. It gave me a powerful mind, a fire in my belly, and a freedom in my spirit. It taught me that life is about taking risks, making mistakes, and eating too much chocolate at times. It's about daring greatly, failing greatly and learning greatly. It's about owning your worth, believing you are good enough and creating space for positive change.

I've written *Yoga Gym* to show you that you have always been beautiful. You have always been good enough. You have always been worthy. Now you're just deciding to be healthier, fitter and stronger. Enjoy the journey.

*Nicola Jane Hobbs*

# Carole's story

## Child carer

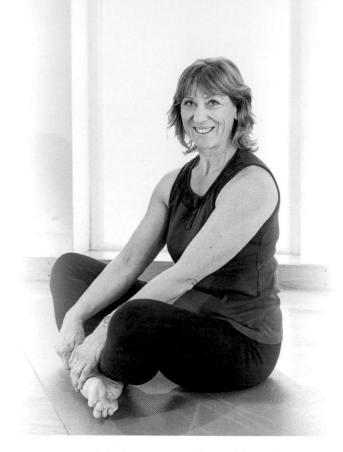

I started yoga 18 months ago as part of a new exercise regime so I could look my best at my daughter's wedding. I wanted to lose a bit of weight, build some muscle to look more toned, and be able to look at my body and be happy with it.

As someone who looks after children for a living, it can be difficult to get to yoga classes, so Yoga Gym is perfect because it can be done anywhere. I do lots of poses throughout the day – in the kitchen, in the living room, and even when I take the children to the park. The kids love joining in too and I think it's brilliant to get them doing yoga at a young age so they can grow up knowing how to look after their bodies.

I love all different types of yoga so really enjoyed the mixture of dynamic flows, challenging yogacises, and calming yin poses in Yoga Gym. My favourite pose is Tree pose (see p. 76) because I can feel it working my core and it helps me to feel focused and balanced. I feel the workouts have really taught me how to listen to my body. This body awareness helped me tune into my appetite and eat healthier and more natural foods so I could get into the best shape possible for my daughter's wedding. On the day of the wedding, some of my family didn't even recognise me because yoga has changed my body so much.

Before I started yoga, I used to be scared of exercising because I had painful knees and hips from years of picking up children. However, since I started regular yoga workouts and have become more aware of my breathing, my posture and the importance of stretching, they are no longer a problem. By strengthening my muscles and increasing my flexibility, Yoga Gym has helped me become pain free.

Yoga has made me mentally stronger too. I know that I can push myself further and get out of my comfort zone in order to grow. I'm now working on headstands and Crow pose (see p. 87), which I thought were impossible when I first started. The breathing techniques I have learnt are also really helpful if I feel stressed or anxious. I know that by breathing properly, I am a calmer person and have a lot more patience. I love how Yoga Gym has helped me find balance in my exercise routine and life. I know the importance of working hard and challenging myself but also make time to nourish myself and relax. For anyone tempted to try yoga my advice would be just do it. Once you start, you will never look back.

# Jim's story

**International athlete and personal trainer**

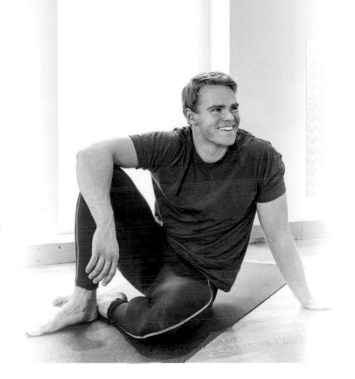

My first experience of yoga occurred when I was travelling in Peru a couple of years ago. I had just left the Marines so wanted to try a completely different type of exercise from the regimented military approach I was used to. I did some yoga every now and then but I ended up focusing on weightlifting and sprinting when I was selected as part of the Great Britain Bobsleigh team last year.

As hobsleigh training became more intense, I noticed my muscles were feeling tight and I felt my athletic performance was being limited by my lack of flexibility, so I began the Yoga Gym plan. Since starting, my passion for yoga has been ignited. It has taught me how important it is to spend time working on my flexibility as well as training for strength and power in order to stay injury free and perform to the best of my ability. I have noticed a huge improvement in my posture and stance, and my balance and co-ordination have improved as I have become more body-aware from performing standing poses. The muscles in the backs of my legs and upper body feel looser and I can perform certain strength and power movements more easily now I have greater mobility in my hips and shoulders.

As a power athlete, my main aim is to be fast and strong. Yoga has helped me to access the power that is needed for sprinting and weightlifting by teaching me how to move mindfully and relax muscles that aren't needed, instead of wasting energy tensing them. My favourite poses are the passive yin poses because they fill me with calm and teach me improvement through relaxation.

One of the biggest things I have learnt from Yoga Gym is that looking after my mind and spirit is just as important, if not more so, than looking after my body. Yoga has had a profound impact on my composure in sport and daily life. As an athlete, I feel more focused and more determined when I train and I now control any pre-competition anxiety using different breathing techniques. In general, I feel happier, calmer and more mindful of my actions.

Being able to do everything in the Yoga Gym plan at home and pick a variation that suits me is great as it supports the training I do at the gym without me having to travel anywhere or buy any equipment.

I love how yoga is non-competitive and I can just enjoy my personal yoga journey – my new goal is to master a handstand! I recommend yoga to all my personal-training clients and would encourage any athlete to have a go at Yoga Gym to support their performance.

# Barbara's story

**Beauty therapist**

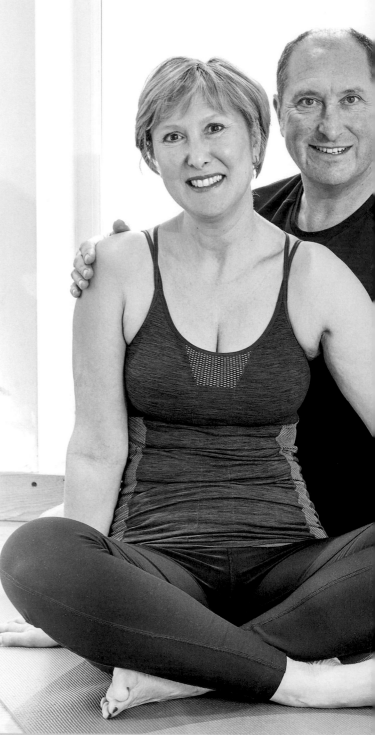

Mark introduced me to yoga after he experienced such positive effects from it on his own health. I had always suffered from lower back pain and spent a lot of time and money visiting medical practitioners looking for a cure. Yoga changed everything and it is now a major part of my life. Since starting the plan, I can now move and bend without any pain and can touch my toes with ease.

I also play tennis, swim and walk, so Yoga Gym complements the other exercise I do really well because it is so versatile. I love being challenged by some of the more strengthening poses and feel my whole body looks more toned. My stomach is more defined too now that I have learnt how to engage my core muscles and use them to stabilise me in standing poses and to support me when I get outside my comfort zone to have a go at headstands and handstands.

As well as the challenge of Yoga Gym, I really look forward to the feeling of relaxation after each session. When I do yin yoga, I feel as though I am talking to my muscles and asking them to release any tension. I find yoga has helped me to switch off and block out any outside noise or stress. If I have trouble sleeping, I use yoga breathing techniques to help.

Yoga has helped me to become a calmer person and taught me things I can apply to my life off the yoga mat. I now listen to my body more and relax if I need to, I can tune into my feelings, and I challenge myself more in lots of areas of my life.

# Mark's story
**Stockbroker**

I discovered yoga about five years ago after being diagnosed with a neurological condition. I used to do a lot of high-impact exercise and competitive sport but had to give those up, so I experimented with various fitness plans to help me manage my condition. When I found yoga, I realised it was the perfect way to keep fit as well as distance my mind from my neurological symptoms by helping me to focus on the present moment.

I find going to regular yoga classes as well as using Yoga Gym as part of my home practice has helped me lose weight and keeps me fit without me having to do a lot of cardiovascular exercise, as I did in the past. Although I miss competitive sport, I find the personal challenges involved in yoga exhilarating. I love dynamic yoga and postures such as Triangle pose (see p. 68), which combines balancing, stretching, twisting and lengthening.

Despite having occasional relapses of my medical condition, yoga has enabled me to regain my flexibility and movement and this has helped with everyday activities. I have a far more relaxed outlook on life and even though I experience a lot of fatigue because of my condition, I know that relaxing properly by using calming breathing techniques will leave me feeling completely invigorated.

For anyone about to embark on Yoga Gym, I would advise you to take time to try out the poses and yogacises so you can understand your limitations, set suitable goals and enjoy your own journey.

# Emily's story
**Project co-ordinator**

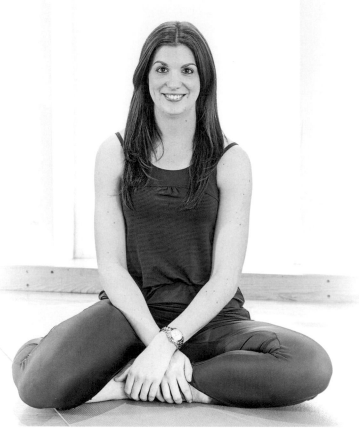

I started yoga a couple of years ago when I was training for a gruelling 300-mile (480km) bike ride. I have suffered from shin splits for years and the pain was limiting my training, but after a few months of doing yoga they virtually vanished. By strengthening the muscles around my shins and in my legs, I can now cycle and run without any pain and have just started training for my first half-marathon.

One of the things I love about yoga is that you can do it just about anywhere – at home, on holiday and even in bed! I work long hours and have a busy social calendar, so Yoga Gym fits into my lifestyle perfectly. It's playful and challenging and I enjoy being able to relax, clear my mind and completely forget about the stress of my job. As well as the Yoga Gym plan, I like being able to choose appropriate poses and yogacises depending on how much time I have and whether I want a tough workout or to relax and restore.

I do a lot of high-impact exercise such as running, spinning and weight training, so I find yoga is a great way to loosen any tight muscles and relieve aches and pains. I love passive yin poses, which I hold for as a long as I can, really tuning into each muscle and allowing it to relax. Regular yoga practice has made me a lot more aware of my posture and breathing too and I'm convinced it has made me taller!

I enjoy the challenge of a strong, dynamic yoga session and can feel my core strength has improved dramatically. I'm much more flexible too and am working towards doing the splits, which is something I couldn't do even as a child.

The main lesson I've learnt from Yoga Gym is to try anything and not to give up – you're never too old to do a headstand! I think it's a great way to challenge yourself and explore what your body is capable of. You can then challenge yourself in a similar way in your everyday life, try things you wouldn't normally attempt, and refuse to give up just because something is difficult to begin with.

Yoga is a big part of my life now. It keeps me slim and fit, does wonders for my stress levels, complements my other training, and is fun and rewarding. I would recommend it to everyone.

# Busting the yoga myths

**'I'm not flexible enough'**

**'I'm not spiritual'**

**'I can't touch my toes'**

**'It's too expensive'**

**'I don't have time'**

As a yoga teacher, I hear many reasons why people are hesitant about trying yoga for the first time. Here are 10 common yoga myths that need to be busted:

## MYTH #1   YOGA IS JUST STRETCHING

Many forms of stretching are involved in yoga in order to improve flexibility, but yoga is about so much more than just stretching. Physically, yoga provides a full-body workout through strengthening postures and challenging flows that build fitness on all levels. Dynamic sequences boost the metabolism to burn fat, whereas passive poses and breathing exercises help to rebalance the nervous system and allow your body to recover quicker between workouts.

## MYTH #2   YOGA IS EASY

A lot of people think that yoga is about sitting cross-legged and 'om'-ing for an hour or two. They think it is easy/boring/not challenging enough. They want the burning muscles, panting breath and sweaty body that comes from a gym session to prove they have worked out hard enough. Though some yoga classes might involve chanting in Lotus pose (see p  100), yoga will certainly give you the muscle burn and sweat too. Yoga will push you way outside your comfort zone without smashing your body to bits.

## MYTH #3   YOU HAVE TO BE ABLE TO TOUCH YOUR TOES

There are no toe-touching prerequisites in yoga and you definitely don't have to be able to twist yourself into a pretzel. How flexible you are depends on various factors, including the elasticity of your tissues, the ability of your muscles to relax, other types of training you are engaging in, your age and your bone structure. Regardless of your current flexibility level, yoga will help you explore your body to find freedom and effortlessness in movement.

## MYTH #4   ONLY WOMEN DO YOGA

There are two common stereotypes in the health and fitness world:

1   Weightlifting is for men.
2   Yoga is for women.

These stereotypes are slowly being broken down as female athletes become a source of inspiration for many young women and male sportsmen do yoga as part of their training. Although there are some physiological differences between men and women that impact on strength and flexibility, men and women are the same species and yoga benefits both equally. So guys, don't be afraid to put down your dumbbells, roll out your yoga mat and break the stereotype.

**MYTH #5**  YOU CAN'T BUILD MUSCLE THROUGH YOGA
Before we begin, for any ladies worried about getting big and bulky, building muscle does not mean building bulk. Building muscle will, however, increase your metabolic rate, reshape your body, shift body fat and overall make you stronger. Many people think you have to lift weights to make your muscles grow (known as hypertrophy). The truth is, your muscles can't tell the difference between a dumbbell or cable machine and your own bodyweight. If you challenge the muscles enough through poses and bodyweight training, your body will be forced to adapt by building more muscle and becoming stronger, leaner and more defined.

**MYTH #6**  YOGA IS RELIGIOUS
Yoga is not a religion – it has no God to worship or rituals you must adhere to. Yoga instead can be seen as a science of life that deals with the body, breath, mind and emotions. Scientists and psychologists are now studying the science of yoga and how it creates measurable changes in the body and brain. Some people may find that as they do yoga they will become more interested in the human spirit, however many people do it purely for health reasons. Regardless of your religion and beliefs, yoga provides an opportunity to improve well-being on physical, mental and spiritual levels.

**MYTH #7**  HOT YOGA IS BEST FOR WEIGHT LOSS
Hot yoga has become increasingly popular with celebrities wanting to stay trim, sports players needing to get lean, and dieters trying to shed a few pounds. The premise is that exercising in the heat forces the body to work harder and therefore burn more calories. However, sweating more doesn't mean you are burning more energy. Research shows hot yoga burns the same amount of calories as normal yoga and any immediate weight loss is likely to be because you are dehydrated. Yoga is a great way to get in shape and is perfectly achievable without any excessive sweating, heat exhaustion or dehydration.

**MYTH #8**   ALL YOGIS ARE VEGETARIAN

Many traditional yogis are vegetarian but a key element of yoga is that it is non-judgemental. Yoga welcomes you as you are – whatever size you are, whatever lifestyle choices you make and whatever diet you follow. Many people find that as they regularly do yoga, they become more in tune with their body, learn what foods make them feel good and move towards a natural diet full of fresh fruit and vegetables. This may mean cutting out meat and dairy as some people thrive on a vegan or vegetarian diet, but it may also mean eating meat and fish when you feel you need it. Focus on eating what makes you feel healthy, strong and energised and not what 'gurus' preach as the only route to enlightenment.

**MYTH #9**   YOGA IS EXPENSIVE

You can spend a fortune on yoga classes and retreats if you want to. Having regular access to a teacher and doing yoga with others is a wonderful social experience but it isn't always affordable or practical. There are plenty of yoga books and free internet resources that will help you develop a strong self-practice at home. Unlike other hobbies and activities, you don't need any equipment for yoga (although a yoga mat is nice to work out on and you can pick these up quite cheaply in local supermarkets and sports shops). The greatest investment you will have to put into yoga is not money – it is time, energy and focus.

**MYTH #10**   YOU HAVE TO DO YOGA
FOR HOURS EVERY DAY

Some traditional styles of yoga do recommend you do yoga six or seven days a week. However, yoga has evolved to fit in with our increasingly busy lives so you can find a style that works for you. This may be a 10-minute practice every morning or a 90-minute session a couple of times a week.

# Yoga Gym benefits

**There is a reason why the popularity of yoga has endured since 500BC. There is a reason why training using bodyweight exercises was adopted by the Spartans and Chinese Warriors over 2500 years ago. There is a reason why using just your body to build your body works. Here are 10 great benefits of using nothing but the power of your body to improve your mental and physical health and fitness:**

#1   FAT-LOSS

Yoga should be at the core of your exercise regime if you want to lose fat. As a form of resistance training, yoga builds muscle, burns fat and boosts the metabolism. It is a myth that steady-state cardio is the best way to burn calories. You don't have to spend hours on a treadmill, cycle hundreds of miles, or puff and pant your way through daily aerobics classes to get lean. In fact, excess aerobic activity can actually cause muscle wastage and decrease your metabolic rate as the body has no demand for extra muscle beyond what is needed to run, swim or cycle.

Whereas aerobic activity predominantly burns calories only when you are exercising, high-intensity yoga oxidises fat for a long time after your workout in order to restore depleted energy and regain homeostasis in the body. Even gentle yoga enhances fat-loss by reducing cortisol levels (the hormone responsible for stress, which is known to increase abdominal fat). And, as well as the direct fat loss, you may find the body awareness you develop through yoga helps you fight food cravings and inspires you to follow a healthy-eating plan.

#2   BUILDS MUSCLE AND STRENGTH

If you want a lean, athletic physique then building muscle is a must. Not only does it create a powerful body shape, but developing muscular strength also has a positive effect on the metabolism of nutrients.  This results in better energy levels and reduced physical and mental fatigue.

You don't need dumbbells to build muscle and get strong. All you need is your body, the will to train hard and the discipline to physically push yourself several times a week. Yoga teaches you to master basic postures and movement patterns before adding resistance and challenging you with more advanced poses and exercises as a form of progressive overload.

One of the key areas yoga builds in terms of muscular strength is the core. This is more than just your abs and obliques (although developing a six-pack is a nice by-product) and involves virtually every muscle in your body. Your core is challenged in every yoga pose to build strength and stability and help you perform better in daily life and other athletic activities.

#3   INCREASES FLEXIBILITY

Flexibility is commonly neglected in many people's fitness regimes. After a hard workout, stretching is often the last thing on your mind as you race to work, rush to pick up the kids or dash home to cook dinner.

Yoga is one way that training for strength and flexibility can be done simultaneously. By using eccentric muscle contractions and moving each joint through its full range of movement, you gain strength without shortening the muscle or compromising mobility.

Flexibility, strength and relaxation are intimately related. As you relax, you will reduce muscular tension and create more length in your tissues. As you create length in your muscles and gain flexibility, you will extend your range of motion to perform more advanced yoga poses. And as you build strength, you will be able to move into these poses more effortlessly and hold them for longer periods of time. This will also enhance your resting posture as you gain muscular balance in terms of the length and strength of your muscles. This can ease back pain (one of the most common reasons people don't exercise) by promoting muscular relaxation and reducing stress on the lower back.

#### #4 IMPROVES OVERALL FITNESS

Yoga achieves results because it uses the whole body in each pose. There's no isolating your medial pectoral muscle on machines that look like something out of a torture chamber or using over-complicated equipment that has no effect on real-world strength. Instead, yoga involves compound movements that are extremely effective for gains in strength, power, balance and coordination. Numerous joints and muscles are engaged in each pose and movement, which builds stability in your core as well as promoting strength improvements throughout the whole body.

Yoga also combines strength and cardio training, meaning you can improve both aerobic and anaerobic fitness in one workout. Dynamic flows and high intensity bodyweight training techniques like Tabatas and Peripheral Heart Action (PHA) Training get your heart rate up, whilst challenging poses encourage muscle and strength development.

#### #5 ANTI-AGING

Weight gain, osteoporosis, cardiovascular disease and poor memory are just some of the common age-related problems that yoga can help to prevent.

From our mid-30s it is common to experience gradual weight gain as our metabolism slows down due to muscle loss. If you continue to eat the same amount, you will end up with a slow and steady increase in weight and body-fat percentage. Add in some yoga to your weekly routine and you will build muscle to keep your metabolic fire ignited. Consistent yoga workouts can also decrease cardiovascular risk factors by lowering cholesterol, blood sugar and stress hormones. The same blood vessels go to the brain as go to the heart, so by getting your heart pumping in a yoga session, you'll also be getting more nutrients to the brain to improve memory.

Bone density is also lost as we age, leading to

conditions such as osteopenia and osteoporosis. As a form of weight-bearing exercise, yoga uses the body as active, living resistance to improve bone health.

### #6   IMPROVES MOOD AND REDUCES STRESS

Stress is endemic in the modern world. Yoga helps to bring balance to our hectic lives. As you do yoga you are also carrying out mindfulness. Focusing on the present moment as you perform each yoga pose or yogacise helps you to let go of any worries or anxieties. This mindfulness is a skill you can then incorporate into other areas of life to reduce stress levels and live more in the now.

The physical poses will help to relieve stress by releasing tension from your body through movement and stretching. Studies have shown that yoga reduces stress physically and psychologically by reducing inflammation, which is linked with depression and anxiety.

Breathing patterns impact on your state of mind, so optimal breathing is a key part of yoga. Short, shallow breaths can be a cause and result of stress. By slowing down your breathing, deepening each inhalation and lengthening each exhalation, you switch off the fight-or-flight response of the sympathetic nervous system and turn on the parasympathetic nervous system, which aids relaxation.

### #7   INCREASES BODY CONFIDENCE

Millions of men and women across the world suffer from feelings of shame about their bodies. Magazines tell us to fight flab, slim down and tone up and the voice in our heads tells us we'll only be good enough when we've got a flat stomach/more toned thighs/bigger biceps…

Yoga can make all the difference: it shifts the focus from what your body looks like to what your body can do. It promotes self-acceptance and creates room for change rather than forcing change upon you through restricted diets and rigid exercise regimes.

Just as yoga can help you to lose fat and build a healthy physique, it can also help you shake off body shame and build a healthy relationship with who you are. You can't hate your way to a healthy body. Yoga is about embracing the body you've got to create the body you want. It is about understanding that you are worthy of self-care through good nutrition and exercise. It is about respecting and looking after your body no matter what your shape or size and enjoying any changes to it on your journey to a healthier way of life.

### #8   PREVENTS INJURY

Injury is one of the main reasons why people stop exercising – and often never start again. Yoga is one of the best ways to prevent aches and pains and the variety of styles mean that it is safe for nearly every exerciser. Simple restorative yoga poses can even be used as a form of rehabilitation from injury.

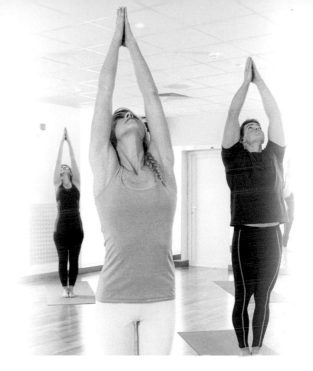

As well as making your body stronger and more supple to reduce your chances of damaging a muscle or connective tissue, yoga also increases body awareness so you are more likely to notice any small niggles or areas of tightness that could lead to bigger injuries in the future. Many athletes now use yoga so they can avoid common sports injuries, such as plantar fasciitis (an overuse injury characterised by pain on the underside of the foot), IT-band syndrome (a common cause of knee pain), hamstring pulls, ankle sprains and rotator cuff tears.

## #9   EFFICIENT AND CONVENIENT

**'I have no time'**

**'I'm too busy'**

**'I hate going to the gym'**

**'There's no one to look after the kids'**

These are all common excuses for not exercising. The truth is, you can do a quick, super-efficient workout in your own home. Yoga yields fantastic fitness gains in a short period of time without the need for any equipment and you don't even have to leave the house. Working out with just your body means there is no waiting for dumbbells or wasting time moving from one exercise machine to the next. There's no organising a babysitter so you can go to the gym or having to book an exercise class two weeks in advance. Yoga eliminates these barriers to exercise so you can get fit at a time that suits you.

## #10   LIMITLESS

Boredom is a barrier to exercise for many of us. If you think healthy living is all about trundling along on a treadmill and living off lettuce leaves then it is likely that your motivation to get fit will dwindle fast. One of the brilliant things about yoga is that the poses and movements are limitless. They can be performed indoors, outdoors, alone, with friends, first thing in the morning, in your lunch hour, close to home, on holiday, in your garden or in your office. Yoga can literally be done anywhere, any time, with anyone, and without any equipment.

It's easy to get stuck in an exercise rut and many people perform the same workout routine for years without making any real progress. Yoga is a refreshing alternative that will challenge the body in a totally different way, so you can break through plateaus and spark progress. The 150 or more variations of yoga poses in this book are just the start of the unlimited variants you can challenge yourself with to reignite passion and purpose in your fitness regime.

# Yoga Gym guidelines

These guidelines have been written so you can make the most out of the plan. They are a bit like the speed limit on a motorway – they get you where you want to go as quickly as you can at the same time as keeping you safe and injury free.

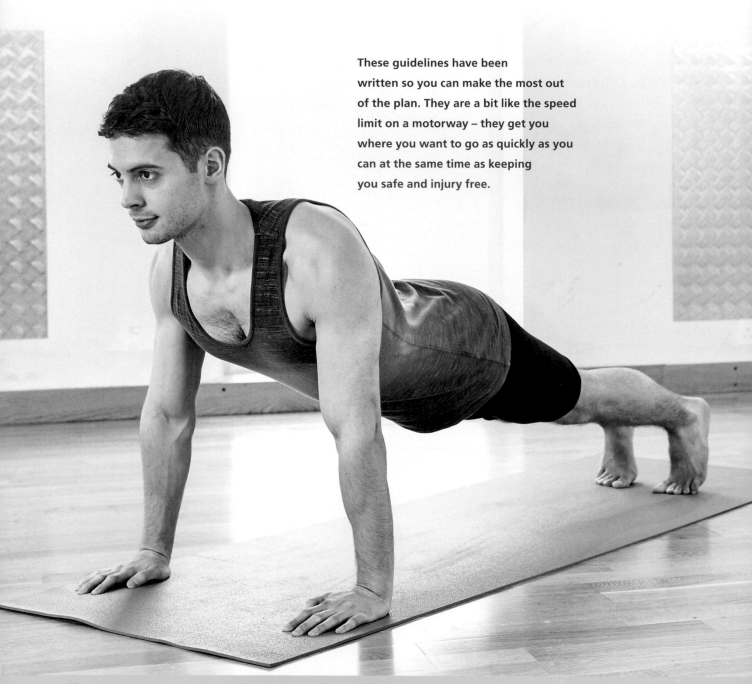

**GUIDELINE #1** YOU ARE THE EXPERT
OF YOUR OWN BODY

The health and fitness world can be a confusing place. We are told that low-carb diets lead to weight loss by some 'experts', whereas other professionals recommend that we load up on starchy carbs to keep trim. Some training plans tell us to work out in the morning on an empty stomach and others propose hitting the gym in the early evening when our nervous system is firing optimally.

In reality, nutritionists know a lot about food, personal trainers know a lot about training, yoga teachers know a lot about yoga, but you know your body better than anyone. You have years of nutrition and exercise expertise from your previous diet and exercise plans. All you need to do is to tap into this knowledge, examine your habits and reflect honestly on what works and what doesn't. Start with some simple questions:

1 What is holding you back from achieving your current health goals?
2 Do you need friends to keep you motivated or do you prefer to keep your fitness goals to yourself?
3 Is exercising inside or outside more enjoyable for you?
4 Do you do better when you focus on how you look or how you feel?
5 Are there any exercises that cause you pain?
6 Which foods leave you feeling energised?
7 What types of food make you feel bloated and lethargic or make you gain body fat?
8 Do you do well with strict diet rules and calorie counting?
9 Do you have any trigger foods that might cause a binge?
10 Does your desire for processed food go away when you eat nutritious food?

Some of our unhealthy eating and exercise habits may have become so engrained that we aren't always conscious of them. Bringing awareness to them like this can sometimes be uncomfortable, but it is only through this awareness that we can become our own expert and reshape our body and our lifestyle.

**GUIDELINE #2**  NO PAIN. ALL GAIN

Pain is a warning signal that something isn't right. That niggle you've been ignoring, the severe tightness in your limbs you overlook and the permanent ache in your joints that you accept as normal are your body's way of telling you that you are doing damage. There is no point in having the physique you are after if your body doesn't actually work.

One of the key lessons you will learn from Yoga Gym is the difference between discomfort and pain. In order to become stronger, leaner and healthier, we need to challenge ourselves and get outside our comfort zone. This is totally different to training through pain and feeling close to collapse at the end of a workout. Exhaustion is not a status symbol. Pain is not acceptable. You may feel strong sensations in some of the postures and some of the workouts may leave you with Delayed Onset Muscle Soreness (DOMS), or that achey feeling the next day or two after exercise, but pain is a signal that the body is injured or in the process of being injured. If a pose causes pain then move out of it slowly, deal with the source of the pain and return to the pose at a later date.

**GUIDELINE #3**  MASTER MOVEMENT

The first goal of Yoga Gym is to help you master movement. The body needs to move the way it is designed to. Unfortunately, society has made it easy for us to be couch potatoes and most of us do not need to move functionally in order to survive. We go from bed to car to office seat to dinner chair to sofa – slouching, slumping and hunching our way through life. This sedentary lifestyle has meant that many of us have forgotten how to move our bodies naturally.

The reason why most of us develop niggles and pains when we start exercising is that we never focus on building a foundation of optimal movement. We launch into park runs without warming up, flail our limbs around in an aerobics session and chuck weights overhead without giving a second thought to how we actually move. Even athletes have a tendency to ignore optimal movement patterns and instead focus on strength, speed and power. This will work for a while, until injuries start occurring as the body becomes more and more out of balance.

Rebuilding optimal movement patterns starts with the most basic and essential of movements – breathing. As you breathe better, you stand better, and as you stand better, you begin to do everyday activities such as lifting and reaching with healthier form. As these optimal movement patterns become engrained, you can progress to an endless array of complex yoga, bodyweight and athletic movements to completely change the way your body performs.

**GUIDELINE #4**  BREAK YOUR OLD RULES

Over time, we slowly build up an array of subconscious exercise rules and habits that can be challenging to break. It may be as simple as always doing cardio before resistance training, always having a bowl of porridge to fuel you through a workout, or never stretching before a weights session. You may have read about these 'rules' in a fitness magazine or heard them in the gym and have convinced yourself that without that bowl of porridge you just won't have the energy for a full session of resistance training.

Yoga Gym is all about trying something new, changing your old routines and mixing up your workouts so you can make progress and look and feel better than ever. Smash your old rules and re-establish what kind of exercise regime suits you and your lifestyle rather than believing in every fitness trend and workout fad that comes along.

## GUIDELINE #5   THERE IS NO MAGIC PILL/SYSTEM/FORMULA

Many of us spend our lives searching for that magic 'thing' that will make us slimmer, leaner, healthier, stronger, more powerful, more muscular, more toned, more energised... We go on quick-fix diets, spend money on specialist supplements and train for hours in the gym to get the body we are after. Most of us never achieve that dream body – we get fed up with the starvation, the restriction, the expense and the sacrifice and move on to find the next miracle cure.

The truth is there is no magic involved when it comes to getting stronger, leaner and healthier. There is no wonder diet. There is no cure-all workout. There is no

hard-and-fast number of repetitions and sets. There is no miracle-working yoga teacher, or personal trainer or coach. There is just hard work, commitment and a balance of self-acceptance and self-improvement.

Eat well, move lots, train hard, listen to your body, remember to relax, enjoy the process and you won't need magic or miracles. No matter what you imagine your limitations to be, no matter what your fitness level is now, no matter what your body currently looks like, if you are willing to undergo change to reshape your body and your life then you will achieve what you want to achieve and become what you want to become. No magic pills or potions, just energy, motivation, and unconditional self-belief.

## GUIDELINE #6   SLEEP IS ESSENTIAL

Sleep is often the first thing that is sacrificed if we're working long hours, managing a house and looking after kids. Commit to a workout plan on top of all of this and few of us get the recommended eight hours a night.

Instead of foregoing sleep, figure out what you spend (and waste) your time on. Browsing social media, mindlessly watching TV and constantly checking our phones are common procrastination tools that eat away at our time. Be conscious of how long you are spending on these activities and figure out whether they are truly nourishing you or if they are merely distractions.

Adequate sleep is essential in order to make the most out of the Yoga Gym plan. It will give your body the opportunity to repair itself and rebuild muscle, to produce the chemicals in your brain that are responsible for mood (e.g. serotonin), and to balance the hormones that affect your appetite to help you achieve a healthy physique.

**GUIDELINE #7**  DO NOT BE AFRAID TO BUILD MUSCLE
One of the main purposes of Yoga Gym is to build muscle. It is not to tone muscle or to sculpt muscle (both are impossible) but to challenge your body enough so that your muscles grow to cope with the demands of the workouts.

For men this means you will experience a large boost in testosterone and growth hormone post-workout, which will help you pack on muscle and grow in size and strength. For females it is a slightly different story. As women have 15–20 times less testosterone than men, there is no need to worry about getting bulky. As a woman, after you train hard only your growth hormone will be elevated. This will help you gain a little muscle (which acts as great ammunition against an age-induced slow metabolism) but its main effects will be fat burning to leave you looking and feeling strong and fit. The more muscle you build through your own hard work and training, the more empowered and body confident you will feel.

**GUIDELINE #8**  EVERY EXERCISE IS A CORE EXERCISE
When most of us think about our core, we think of flat stomachs and rippling abs. Although a strong core and six-pack often go hand in hand, core strength has far more benefits than helping us look good in our swimming gear. Our core underpins everything we do in daily and sporting life. Whether you're doing a yoga pose, mopping the floor or putting on your socks, all the necessary movements involve your core.

Think of your core as a link between your upper and lower body – including your diaphragm, gluteal muscles, pelvic floor and everything besides your arms and legs. By building stability in these areas, you can crank up the power you generate in your limbs, improve flexibility by creating a stable pelvis and help prevent falls, injuries and lower back pain. Many of our limits in flexibility are due to lack of core strength (which no amount of stretching will help). For example, a common cause of tight hamstrings is an unstable pelvis that is the result of a weak core. This means the hamstrings do work they are not designed to do in an attempt to create stability. This leads to the hamstrings overworking, fatiguing and straining, causing sub-optimal performance and even injury. If you want to improve mobility in your limbs, first focus on building strength in your core.

**GUIDELINE #9**  HAVE FUN
In our achievement-orientated world, we seem to think that everything worthwhile involves pain and suffering. Unless we are sweating, crawling or shaking at the end of a workout it must not have been effective. Wrong.

Just because the process of completing a workout or reaching a goal happens to be fun does not mean it has any less value than something we may find more difficult or time-consuming.

Working hard and having fun are not dichotomies. If you want to get fitter and healthier then you might as well enjoy the process. Sometimes all it takes is an attitude shift. If you hate exercise, rather than avoid it, make it fun. Work out with friends, do yoga to your favourite pop songs or exercise naked!! Fun and excellence go hand in hand – treat your workouts as play time and you will be amazed by the results.

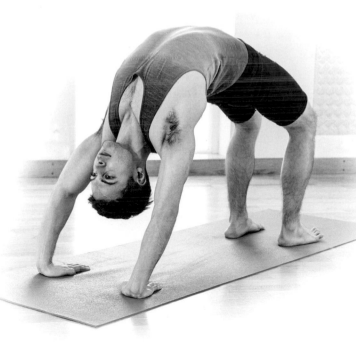

**GUIDELINE #10**   BEING HEALTHY IS NOT A COMPETITION

This is your journey. You don't have to meet anyone else's expectations. You don't have to compare yourself to anyone else in order to determine your own self-worth. You want to move forwards. To become stronger, leaner, more flexible, to learn how to listen to your body, to become more athletic, more body confident, more empowered. Yoga is not a race. It will take time because there is no finish line. There is no 'perfect'.

There is no winner and loser when it comes to Yoga Gym. You are different from everyone else reading this book and cannot be compared to anyone. The unity that comes from yoga frees us from a competitive state of mind and unites us with a supportive community in which each person is on their own journey towards living a healthier life.

It doesn't matter if your best friend can do the splits or if your partner can do more push-ups than you can. Day-to-day improvements are a more meaningful measure of progress than who beats whom. We all work out and do yoga for reasons that are unique to us. We might be aiming to be strong and supple, healthy and happy, or powerful and peaceful. We may want to be able to do a Handstand, or hold a Plank, or just dedicate some time to ourselves each day. When you're doing yoga, forget about comparing yourself to anyone else, forget about comparing your body and your fitness levels to yesterday or two weeks ago or 10 years ago, and focus on embracing your workout one open-minded breath at time.

# Yoga Gym diet

**Yoga Gym is not just about the 30–50 minutes you spend exercising during each workout. Just as you commit to your workouts, you need to commit to nourishing yourself properly every day.**

Diet comes from the Latin word 'diaeta' meaning 'day's journey'. It is only in the modern world that we have begun to associate 'diets' with restriction and semi-starvation. The Yoga Gym diet follows the original meaning of the word by stepping away from strict food regimes and offering you guidance you can implement every day. No rules. No restrictions. Just principles to guide you.

**PRINCIPLE #1  KNOW YOURSELF**

Nutrition is pretty simple but we insist on making it complicated. There are various diets that claim to be the best. From Paleo and vegan to Atkins and Ayurveda, each has its own theory and success stories to support its effectiveness. This highlights how different diets work for different people. We may feel great after eating a good-quality steak whereas our friend may feel better being fuelled by plants.

Just as you listen to your body at the gym or on your yoga mat, so you must listen to your body at the dinner table. See if any foods make you feel bloated and lethargic and avoid them. Find out which foods nourish you, energise you and satisfy you and eat more of them.

If you try and follow the advice in every diet book you will end up in a state of nutritional confusion. Instead, learn to tune into your body's satiety signals and eat what makes you feel good. You are the expert of your own body – listen to it.

**PRINCIPLE #2  DRINK MORE WATER**

Forget superfoods. Forget expensive supplements. Water is the most important element of a healthy diet. Every day we need to drink at least 2 litres (1.75 quarts) of water to replace the amount we lose through urinating, breathing and sweating. If we are dehydrated by just 1 per cent our sport and exercise performance is impaired, and if we have water losses of 2.5 per cent our body's capacity to perform high-intensity exercise can cut virtually in half.

Keeping hydrated improves your fitness by keeping your core temperature and heart rate low so you can push yourself further, and it will help you lose fat by keeping your metabolic rate high. Optimal hydration also helps your liver work more effectively to flush out toxins that have been released from your tissues through twisting and stretching.

### PRINCIPLE #3   EAT REAL FOOD
The quality of your food is just as important as the quantity. Your body responds totally differently to a 200-kcalorie chocolate bar than it does to 200 kcalories of fresh vegetables.

Eating whole foods (foods that are unprocessed and unrefined) is about going back to eating foods that the human body is designed to eat. Millions of years ago, humans lived off just a few things – meat, fish, eggs, fruit, vegetables, nuts, seeds and legumes. These are the foods that fuel your body most effectively. They are the most nutrient-dense, free from any artificial ingredients, readily available, affordable, and taste good. A general guide for eating real food is that if you can't grow it, pick it, kill it or dig it up from the ground then don't eat it. And if you can't pronounce it then certainly don't eat it – just look at the ingredients list on a 'healthy' snack bar and you will probably find 'polyglycerol

polyricinoleate', 'azodicarbonamide' or some other unpronounceable additive or preservative. Avoid it.

If you need a snack, instead of choosing a processed cereal bar because it is marketed as 'healthy' or 'low fat', go for an apple and a handful of nuts. Your body (and your bank balance) will thank you for it.

### PRINCIPLE #4   FEED YOUR MUSCLES
'Eat less and exercise more' is the traditional weight-loss advice. In theory it makes sense – cut calories from food and burn calories through exercise. But in reality the human body is far more complex. If you under-eat, not only will weight loss be ineffective in the long term but you will impact on numerous hormones including oestrogen (important for female fertility), leptin (regulates appetite), cortisol (stress hormone) and thyroid hormones, which will result in a slow metabolism. Self-starvation may even give you higher body fat levels as you start burning lean tissue for fuel.

Weighing scales bear little relevance to your health. Losing 3kg (6½lb) of fat may be beneficial but losing 3kg (6½lb) of muscle certainly won't be. It's far better to eat enough to feed your muscles, lose fat slowly and keep it off long term – and that may mean eating more (shock, horror!) of the right foods to reach your goals.

**HOW TO CALCULATE YOUR BASAL METABOLIC RATE**

A COMMONLY USED CALCULATION TO WORK OUT HOW MUCH YOU NEED TO EAT IS THE HARRIS-BENEDICT EQUATION. FIRST YOU NEED TO CALCULATE YOUR BASAL METABOLIC RATE (BMR) – THE ENERGY YOU USE AT REST:

**MEN**:
Basic Metabolic Rate = 66.5 + (13.8 x weight in kg) + (5 x height in cm) – (6.75 x age in years)

**WOMEN**:
655 + (9.5 x weight in kg) + (1.85 x height in cm) – (4.8 x age in years)

Once you've calculated your BMR you need to multiply it according to your activity level to determine your daily calorie needs:

<u>BMR</u> x 1.2 = sedentary
<u>BMR</u> x 1.375 = lightly active
(light exercise 1–3 days per week)
<u>BMR</u> x 1.55 = moderately active
(moderate exercise 3–5 days per week)
<u>BMR</u> x 1.725 = very active
(heavy exercise 6–7 days per week)
<u>BMR</u> x 1.9 = extremely active
(heavy exercise daily and a physical job)

If you want to lose weight in a sustainable way, general recommendations suggest that you reduce your calorie intake by 10 per cent of your daily calorie needs. Reducing your calorie intake by more than this won't necessarily lead to faster results but will slow down your metabolism and leave you feeling tired and grumpy. If you want to gain weight by building muscle, experiment by taking on an extra 10 per cent of calories above your daily calorie requirements, from real foods, when doing regular resistance training.

These calculations are a very rough guide. Your body is not a computer and how much you need to eat depends on your body composition, your exercise experience, the quality of food you eat and your time of the month (men have a hormone cycle too!). Use the equations here to make sure you're eating enough, and as you become tuned into your hunger and satiety levels shift the focus back to listening to your body and eating intuitively.

**PRINCIPLE #5**  EMBRACE THE POWER OF PROTEIN
Protein is an essential macronutrient that helps with the growth and repair of the body. It is made up of amino acids – the building blocks of life. The body can make some of these amino acids itself but others, such as tryptophan and leucine, we need to get from our diets.

Good sources of protein include meat, fish, eggs and dairy products. If, like many traditional yogis, you follow a vegetarian or vegan diet, focus on sourcing your protein from green vegetables, quinoa, nuts, beans, lentils and tofu.

During an exercise plan it is especially important we eat enough protein to support the functioning of the body and preserve and build muscle. The basic recommendation for protein intake to prevent deficiency is 0.8g per kg (or 0.36g per lb) of bodyweight. It is common for athletes to eat around 2g of protein per 1kg (2.2lb) of bodyweight. For example, a 55kg (121lb) female athlete may eat around 110g (4oz) protein per day whereas an 85kg (187lb) male athlete would need about 170g (6oz). As a guide, aim for 30–35 per cent of your total energy intake to come from protein and make sure you consume a protein-heavy meal after each workout.

### PRINCIPLE #6  DON'T FEAR FAT

Many people associate eating fat with becoming fat. Food manufacturers have jumped on our fat phobia and fooled us into believing their fat-free products are good for us. The contradiction of 'reduced-fat peanut butter' and 'fat-free cooking oil' highlights our nutritional confusion. The truth is, fat is an essential part of our diet and plays a crucial role in weight management, the absorption of key vitamins, and boosting our immunity. It is important, however, to distinguish between the different types of fat.

Unsaturated fats can be divided into:

**Monounsaturated:** These are healthy fats that are found in avocados, nuts and olive oil. The body uses these fats for energy and to make hormones without raising cholesterol levels.

**Polyunsaturated:** Omega 3 and Omega 6 are the main categories of polyunsaturated fats. These are healthy essential fats that we need to get in our diet from foods such as grass-fed meat, fish, eggs and nuts. Aim to eat oily fish such as salmon or mackerel three times a week or supplement your diet with a good-quality fish oil.

**Trans:** This is an unnatural and unhealthy type of fat found in many processed foods. Trans fats are formed when a liquid fat is artificially made into a solid via hydrogenation. This is the kind of fat you find in margarines and low-calorie spreads and has been linked to high cholesterol and heart conditions.

Saturated fats were demonised for years as unhealthy and artery-clogging and deemed the cause of obesity. But tides have turned and countries such as Sweden are now recommending a diet higher in saturated fats because of its potential benefits to reduce body fat, lower blood sugar and improve good cholesterol. This doesn't mean you can eat as much fat as you like. Not every source of saturated fat is healthy. Avoid processed foods and stick with natural sources such as grass-fed red meat, eggs and coconut oil.

**PRINCIPLE #7** GET CLUED UP ON CARBS

Cutting back on carbs is a common way to lose weight, but cut back too much and you could make yourself vulnerable to anxiety, depression and impaired cognitive function. Low-carb diets have become popular over the last decade with varying degrees of success. Having a moderate amount of carbs in your diet (up to 30–50 per cent of your total energy intake) will provide a key source of energy, fibre, and vitamins and minerals.

Carbohydrates can broadly be divided into fruit and vegetables, grains, and legumes. When picking fruit and vegetables, go for those with the deepest colours (for example, choosing spinach over iceberg lettuce) because they contain the best quality and quantity of vitamins and minerals. When choosing grains, go for slow-digesting wholegrain varieties such as rice, sweet potatoes and oats, and avoid eating processed carbohydrates on a regular basis even if they have been fortified with nutrients. This doesn't mean faster-acting carbohydrates such as bananas and white potatoes are off the menu, just time them so you eat them straight after a workout to replenish glycogen stores in your muscles and help synthesise protein.

Be aware of how you feel after eating bread or other products containing gluten. Modern wheat is different from traditional varieties, leaving some people sensitive to gluten (if you suffer from bloating,

migraines, mood issues or joint inflammation you may be one of them). Also avoid added sugars in food, especially 'high fructose corn syrup' because of its links with diabetes and metabolic disease.

To put it simply, eat carbs that are as close to their natural form as possible to refuel after a workout and when you feel you need more energy.

**PRINCIPLE #8** PARTY SMART – ALCOHOL AND EATING OUT

Healthy eating doesn't mean taking a lunchbox full of chicken and broccoli to your friend's dinner party or sticking to a plate of lettuce leaves when eating out. Be guided by the other principles of healthy eating and allow for a little flexibility. Most restaurants now offer healthy options and are happy to substitute some food items on their menu for more nutritious alternatives. Ask to replace your French fries with new potatoes, to have any creamy dressings served on the side of salads, and swap mayonnaise for salsa or hummus. Be aware of anything that is fried and order extra vegetables as a side dish to boost your nutrient intake. If you really fancy a dessert or are meeting friends for coffee and cake then opt to share and ask for an extra spoon. Be aware of how much you are drinking too. Cafe-style hot drinks such as lattes and hot chocolate can contain more than 500 kcalories, so opt instead for an Americano or black coffee.

Alcohol is empty calories and offers no nutrition. A large glass of wine averages 190 kcalories, a pint of beer contains 220 kcalories, and some creamy cocktails reach more than 650 kcalories. It's great to party once every so often but drink responsibly and intersperse alcoholic drinks with water to keep you hydrated.

## PRINCIPLE #9 EXPERIMENT WITH HEALTHY SUBSTITUTIONS

Many traditional comfort foods and snacks can be replaced with healthier alternatives, which are simple enough to buy or make. For example, if you are going dairy-free, most supermarkets now stock almond and coconut milk. If you want something a bit lighter than mashed potato, try mashed cauliflower. If you want a gluten-free alternative to spaghetti, shred a butternut squash into strips. And if you're craving ice cream, then keep some chopped-up bananas in the freezer to blend into a delicious frozen treat when a hot day strikes.

If you're a foodie and enjoy baking then you can take healthy eating to a whole new level by transforming your favourite recipes so that as well as tasting good they make you feel good too. Beetroot is a great addition to brownie recipes, date paste can replace sugar in most cake recipes, and you can make delicious chocolate mousses out of nothing more than puréed avocados, agave syrup or honey and unsweetened cacao or cocoa powder.

## PRINCIPLE #10 STOP AIMING FOR THE PERFECT DIET

At the end of the day you can only eat so well. The stress caused by trying to maintain a 'perfect' diet will outweigh any positive effects of following that diet. It is the more subtle elements of your lifestyle and mindset that will determine long-term well-being. Just as we cultivate physical flexibility through doing yoga, we can build flexibility into our diet.

Many people find it helpful to use the 80:20 rule as they transition into a new way of healthy eating – eating fresh, natural, whole foods 80 per cent of the time and allowing yourself the freedom to have the odd slice of cheesecake or glass of wine 20 per cent of the time. For example, if you eat three meals a day, that makes up 21 meals a week. If you follow the 80:20 rule, this encourages you to stick to whole foods for 17 meals and gives you greater flexibility for four of them. This breaks the diet mentality of 'good' and 'bad' foods and encourages you to live a balanced lifestyle of health, fun and happiness.

Rather than aiming to have the perfect diet, aim to have the freedom to eat. When you let go of restriction and take a more relaxed view of nutrition, you will find that you will want to eat what you need, rather than feeling you need to eat what you want.

# Yoga Gym mind

Yoga Gym is about more than the workouts that you do and the food you eat. Yoga Gym is about nurturing a strong and powerful mind that will keep you motivated in your workouts and inspired, passionate and content in everyday life. The 10 principles of a Yoga Gym mind are taken from traditional elements of yoga known as the 'yamas' and the 'niyamas'. These are values, guidelines and commitments that focus our efforts and allow us to be at peace with our body, our diet, our training, ourselves, our family and our world.

**VALUE #1   NON-HARM**

Yoga Gym is not about using exercise to punish ourselves for eating an extra serving of cake. It is not about starving ourselves because we don't believe our current body shape is good enough. It is not about judging ourselves if we can't do a yoga pose or complete a workout. Yoga Gym is about training, eating and living with compassion. It is about accepting our body, learning how far we can push ourselves, and knowing that sometimes we need to take a step back and relax.

It is common to see gym-goers and athletes forcing their bodies to do exercises they are not ready to do – potentially harming their body and their self-esteem. By respecting yourself and taking the time to train and relax without self-criticism, self-judgement or self-harm, you will create a stronger version of you that you can share with those you love.

**VALUE #2   TRUTHFULNESS**

Yoga Gym is designed for everyone – man or woman, newbie or experienced yogi, athlete or first-time exerciser. Because of this, there will be some poses and yogacises that you will find easy and some that you find more challenging. Being truthful about your own capabilities in the workouts is crucial for preventing injury and exhaustion. The yoga poses and yogacises come with variations for all levels, so be honest about which one suits you. By not deceiving ourselves about our abilities, we can transform any weaknesses into strengths.

**VALUE #3   SELF-SUFFICIENCY**

If you look around a gym, an athletics meet or a military training session, those who are the strongest, leanest and most powerful are those who are training alone. They have the knowledge, focus and commitment to stick to a training plan until they get the desired results. Working out with a friend or in a group fitness class can be fun, but it can also throw up excuses not to exercise (e.g. if your regular class gets cancelled or your friend drops out as your training partner). Only you know your body, your goals and your time commitments. If you want to be successful in the long term you need to build independence into your training.

**VALUE #4   WISE USE OF ENERGY**

There are times during the day when we feel lively, focused, creative, energetic and persistent, and there are times where we feel drained, droopy, lazy and irritated. These variations in energy levels are usually pretty predictable, so aim to match the tasks on your to-do list with your energy level at that time of the day. There is no point in doing your filing or making phone calls when your energy is its peak if it means that you will then struggle through a Yoga Gym session when all you want to do is chill out. It might be helpful to find a few energy boosters (e.g. a walk around the block, a cold shower or an upbeat music track) you can use for those days when you are feeling weary when it comes to workout time.

During your workout, make sure you are 100 per cent

focused on each pose or yogacise so you aren't wasting physical energy by engaging unnecessary muscles or frittering mental energy by letting your mind wander.

## VALUE #5   FREEDOM FROM 'SHOULD'-ING

Sometimes we try so hard to be perfect in our training that we end up grasping for the ideal diet and the best exercise regime and miss the essence of our workout. We create ideas in our mind of what our body 'should' look like, or what poses and yogacises we 'should' be able to do, or how much fat we 'should' lose or muscle we 'should' gain. There is a difference between a burning desire to train and clinging to the results we expect of ourselves. When you let go of the 'shoulds', stop measuring the distance you have yet to travel, and do your best in each Yoga Gym workout, you are able to focus on every pose, save yourself from injury caused by pushing yourself too far, too fast, and allow yourself to grow stronger.

## VALUE #6   PURITY

A key element of traditional yoga is having a pure body and a pure mind. This isn't about deprivation or holiness, but is expressed by making conscious choices about the foods we eat, the exercises we do, the relationships we have and what we do and don't want in life. Each Yoga Gym workout helps to purify the body through twists, flows and movements that release toxins. The nutritional advice in this book supports the health and purity of the body by recommending real foods that are full of nutrients, while the breathing techniques and meditative elements in Part 2 contribute to a pure mind that is free from worries, fears and anxieties.

## VALUE #7   CONTENTMENT

For most of us, being content with who we are, what we look like, what we have and what we do is tough. There will always be people out there who we see as being more beautiful, more successful, more talented, with better bodies, bigger houses and faster cars. Being content is about being satisfied with what we have and who we are. This is not the same as complacency and allowing our fitness to decline, our motivation to dwindle and our personal growth to stagnate. Contentment is about finding the balance between unconditional self-acceptance and continual self-improvement. It is about recognising where we are in each yoga pose and how many push-ups/squats/crunches we can do, and aiming to progress without criticising where we are now. When we stop pushing and pulling for change and accept ourselves for who we are, we create the space to become stronger, leaner, healthier and happier.

## VALUE #8   SELF-DISCIPLINE

Self-discipline is not about punishment. Self-discipline is

having enough respect for yourself to make choices that nourish your well-being. This includes going to bed at a reasonable time rather than mindlessly watching television, refraining from drinking too much alcohol at a party, and ignoring the excuses that stop you from doing a workout. Just as failure and quitting become a habit, so does self-discipline. The more disciplined you are in one part of your life, the more willpower you will have in other areas. Yoga Gym gives you a plan to follow to help you reach your goal of being stronger, losing fat, mastering handstands, or learning more about yoga, so all you need is the self-discipline to follow it through.

## VALUE #9   SELF-REFLECTION

Developing self-awareness is essential if you want to live a healthier and happier life. Being aware of our strengths gives us confidence, inspiration and satisfaction and only by recognising our weak points can we improve and grow. Spending time reflecting and increasing your awareness may be uncomfortable to start with, as you become conscious of unhealthy habits and open your eyes to the odd chink in your armour, but habits can be made healthy and chinks can be patched up. Only by being conscious of these weaknesses can we generate the action needed to change. Give yourself 10 minutes of 'think time' every day to reflect on your training, your diet, your body, your relationships, your work and your social life. Bring your awareness to what makes you happy, what you are grateful for and what you would like to change.

## VALUE #10   MEANING

We make meaning through the attention we express in our actions. It is therefore essential that you bring meaning to your workouts and look at the bigger picture rather than just doing push-ups with no thought. You may have a long-term goal to lose weight so you can play football with your kids, to reduce stress levels so you are more patient with your friends, or to get more flexible so you can make the school athletics team. Some people find it helpful to set themselves an intention at the start of each workout so they can let go of cluttered thoughts and worries and bring their full attention to their training. When we bring meaning to every experience, we find interest and enjoyment in what may once have been boring and meaningless. When we hold Warrior Pose we feel the strength in our thighs; when we do push-ups we experience the power in our arms; when we eat a salad, we taste its freshness; and when we take time to really look at our body in the mirror, we see and value its health, strength and unique beauty.

# Equipment & extras

**The beauty of Yoga Gym is that all you need is your body, your mind and your breath – no weights, no machines, no excuses.**

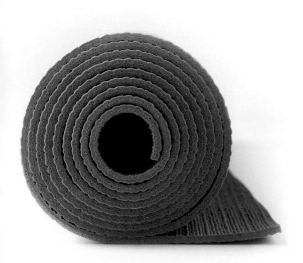

**YOGA EQUIPMENT**

YOU HAVE ALL YOU NEED WITHIN YOU FOR THE YOGA GYM PLAN, BUT THERE ARE A FEW BITS OF EQUIPMENT YOU MIGHT FIND HELPFUL:

### YOGA MAT

A yoga mat will provide you with a non-slip surface and a bit of cushioning. The edges of the mat also serve as a good reference point so you can make sure you are in alignment in each pose. Manduka and Liforme make great yoga mats or you can pick one up in most supermarkets or sports shops and online.

### YOGA BLOCKS AND STRAP

Blocks and straps are a wise investment if you feel you have particularly tight muscles or you want to really focus on increasing your flexibility. You can improvise by using cushions or piles of books instead of yoga blocks and by using a standard belt instead of a yoga strap, but you can pick both up fairly cheaply in sports shops and online.

### MUSIC PLAYLIST

Some days it can be great fun to do yoga to music and other times it's lovely to train in silence. It's a good idea to create a playlist of some of your favourite motivating music to keep you energised throughout the practice. Go for some faster upbeat tunes for the more dynamic parts of the session and some gentle, peaceful tracks to help you relax.

## BODY

The military, martial artists and Olympic athletes have known for years that the body is the greatest piece of fitness equipment on earth. Yoga Gym uses the body as an active, living, moving dumbbell. Using only your bodyweight provides you with a chance to observe your body, how you stand and move, and whether there are any areas of pain or discomfort. Once you get to know and accept your body as it is, you can embrace its power to become healthier and stronger and create the kind of physique you want without risking injury.

## MIND

There may be times during Yoga Gym workouts when your body aches, your stomach knots, and all you can think about is giving up. This is why it is so important to focus on building a powerful mind alongside a strong body. It is only in the modern Western world that we have divided the mind and body into two separate entities. Traditional yoga approaches treat the human form as a single 'bodymind'. Yoga Gym follows this approach. As you improve your flexibility and release tightness from your muscles, you may also experience an emotional release and find yourself become more open-minded. As you lose fat and create a healthy physique, you may also lose any worries and stresses. And as you build physical strength you will experience focus, commitment and self-motivation on a whole new level.

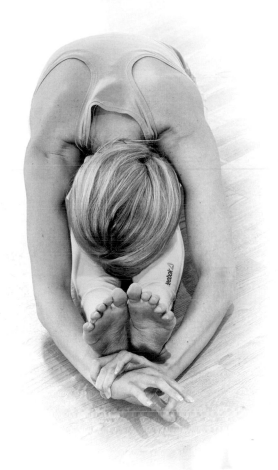

## BREATH

The breath is the most underused tool in exercise and in daily life. How we breathe affects everything from the health of our spine and our mood to our performance on a football pitch. Ancient yogis found that breathing techniques (traditionally known as 'pranayama') can bring the body and mind into a harmonious state by harnessing 'prana' – also known as 'qi' or 'chi' in Chinese medicine, and named 'bioenergy' in quantum mechanics. The breathing exercises in Part 2 will teach you different ways to use the power of your breath to get the most out of your workouts, improve the function of your muscular, circulatory, digestive, nervous and immune systems, and leave you feeling energised, calm and relaxed.

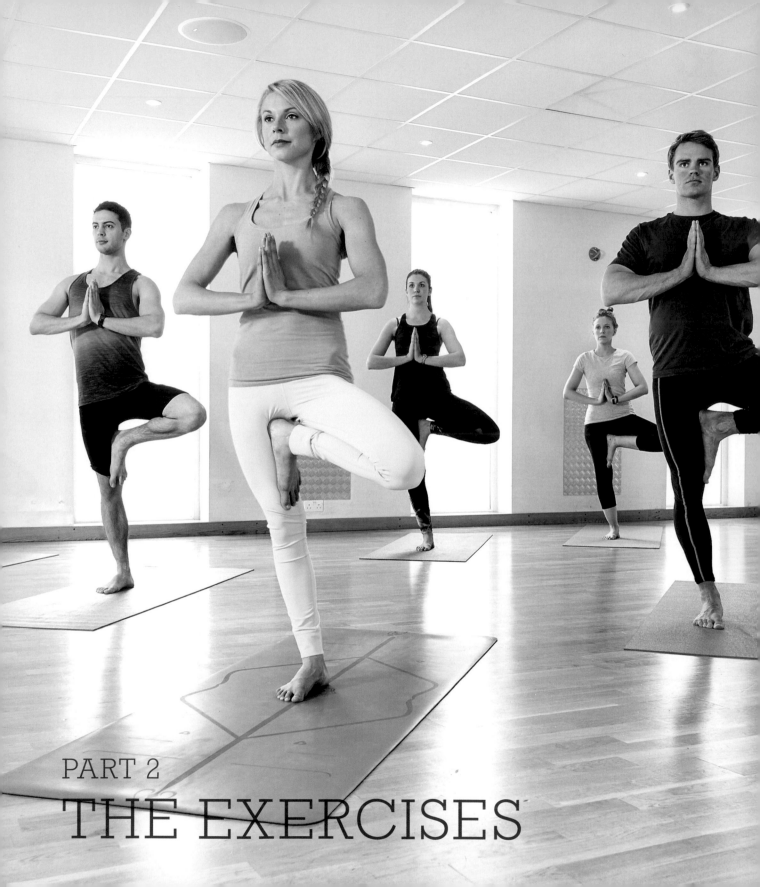

PART 2

# THE EXERCISES

# Key concepts

**The Yoga Gym exercises and plan are generally suitable for all ages and abilities, but there are still a few safety points you should take note of:**

- If you have any illnesses or injuries that could be exacerbated by physical activity, or you are pregnant, then seek advice from your doctor before increasing your exercise levels.
- The yoga poses and yogacises are designed to challenge you, but if you feel dizzy, faint or are in pain at any point during your workout, stop exercising and seek medical advice.
- Make sure you exercise in a safe space with enough room for you to move your arms and legs around without hitting anything.
- Read over the description for each yoga pose and yogacise before beginning your workout to ensure you have the correct form and good posture.
- Drink water regularly throughout your workout to keep hydrated.
- If in doubt about poses, yogacises or workouts then you can contact me via my website at www.YogaGymRevolution.com

# The Stabilising Sequence

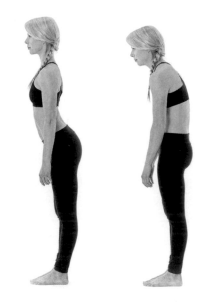

POOR POSTURE: *anterior (l) and posterior (r)*

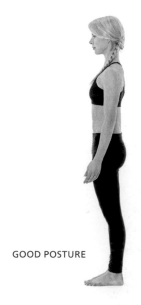

GOOD POSTURE

An exercise is only as good as the posture in which you perform it.

Before you attempt to manoeuvre your body into yoga poses it is important that you know how to stabilise your spine. Optimal posture is the foundation of optimal flexibility, so we must create stability in the core before we can build mobility in the limbs.

If you take a moment to look at people in the street, or in your workplace or even in your house, you'll probably notice that they are slumping with their back rounded and shoulders falling forwards. This is a default position for many of us but it is far from healthy and often results in tension headaches, back pain, fatigue, poor breathing, and even slipped discs. The good news is that you can re-teach your body optimal posture through a simple three-step technique called the Stabilising Sequence.

Using the Stabilising Sequence whenever you are standing or before you sit down or perform a yoga pose or yogacise will bring your body into alignment and stabilise your spine in a neutral position. And, just as any habit becomes automatic over time, this stable neutral posture will eventually become your default position.

Start by trying out the three-stage Stabilising Sequence somewhere you can look side-on in a mirror and notice how your posture changes:

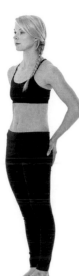

**1 SQUEEZE YOUR BUM:** Engaging the muscles in your bottom (the gluteal muscles) will set your pelvis in a neutral position. First, make sure your feet are parallel to each other. Squeeze your bottom as hard as you can and imagine lengthening your tailbone and tucking it under. This will tilt your pelvis into a healthy position and bring your spine into alignment.

**2 BRACE YOUR BELLY:** To make the spine more stable we brace our belly to lock the pelvis in place and create intra-abdominal pressure. To begin with, aim to align your ribcage over your pelvis to prevent your ribs from popping out. Brace your belly by imagining that someone is about to punch you in the stomach and exhale forcefully to firm your stomach (this is not the same as sucking in your belly).

**3 ROLL YOUR SHOULDERS BACK AND DOWN:** The final step creates stability in your shoulders and lifts the chest forwards. Start by rolling your shoulders up and backwards and then let them fall down your back so your arms dangle comfortably by your sides with your palms facing

forwards. Finally, draw your head back so your neck is in line with the rest of your vertebrae and balancing effortlessly on the top of your spine.

A quick cue to remember the Stabilising Sequence is: **1. Bum. 2. Belly. 3. Back.**

Aim to perform the Stabilising Sequence at various times throughout the day and before you do each pose or yogacise in your workout so you engrain a stable position in your routine. At first, it can be challenging to keep your shoulders back at the same time as squeezing your bottom, but as both your body-awareness and mind-muscle connections improve, slouching and slumping will become a thing of the past.

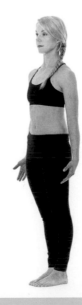

# Healthy Wrist Sequence

A common complaint when people start doing yoga or bodyweight training is tenderness in the wrists. This isn't anything to worry about and any discomfort will disappear as your wrists become stronger.

When doing poses and yogacises that require you to take a significant amount of weight on your hands, such as Plank (see p. 84), Crow (see p. 87), and Push-ups (see p. 122), try digging the tips of your fingers into the ground to activate the muscles in your forearms and take any strain off your wrists. Also focus on pressing down with the knuckles where your fingers join your palms instead of taking all of the weight in the heel of your hand.

If you're feeling mild pain in your wrists or you feel the joints are particularly weak or tight, then have a go at doing the following sequence before your workout or at various times throughout the day:

**1 WRIST CIRCLES:** Slowly rotate your wrists in a circular motion for 1–2 minutes, making sure you change direction often.

**2 PRAYER HANDS:** Press your palms firmly together in front of your chest and hold for 1–2 minutes.

**3 REVERSE PRAYER:** Press the backs of your hands together in front of your chest with your fingers pointing down and hold for 1–2 minutes.

**4 WRIST DANCE:** Begin on all fours in Table Top (see p. 78) and turn your hands upside down so the backs of your hands are on the floor with your fingers facing you. Bring your fingers to face inwards with your palms on the floor, then turn them over with your fingers facing outwards, and keep turning them for 1–2 minutes, so that your palms face up and down, and your fingers face inwards, outwards, forwards and backwards.

# Types of exercise

**There are five different types of exercises in the Yoga Gym plan:**

**1 BREATHING EXERCISES:** Breathing is the earliest form of movement. We cannot move optimally and increase our flexibility and strength unless we are breathing optimally.

**2 YANG POSES:** These are challenging poses that are designed to strengthen the muscles, tone the limbs and improve flexibility using active stretching.

**3 FLOWS:** These are breath-synchronised movements that warm up the body and prepare the nervous system for exercise.

**4 YOGACISES:** These combine traditional yoga poses with bodyweight exercises to improve fitness on all levels, including aerobic fitness, strength, flexibility, power and agility.

**5 YIN POSES:** These are passive poses held for longer periods of time to encourage the body and mind to relax and improve flexibility by creating slack in the muscles.

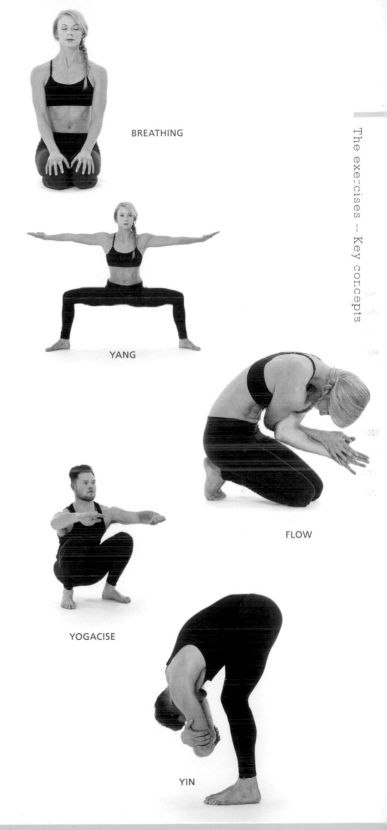

BREATHING

YANG

FLOW

YOGACISE

YIN

# Breathing exercises

**Breathing is the most basic form of movement. It is the first movement we make when we are born and has a huge impact on our posture, flexibility, strength and mood. Breathing is an automatic process so we usually think very little about it, which means many of us are not breathing optimally. By paying our breath a little bit of attention we can completely change how we stand, move and feel.**

## BENEFITS OF BREATHING EXERCISES

- Trains the body to use its entire range of breathing apparatus by paying attention to lower, middle and upper parts of each breath
- Strengthens the diaphragm
- Increases oxygen supply to the blood to power the limbs, organs and muscles
- Increases awareness of where you hold tension in the body and how to release it
- Empties the lungs completely to remove waste products
- Massages internal organs and improved digestion
- Improves posture
- Helps to reduce anxiety
- Switches the body from fight-or-flight mode to a relaxed resting and digesting mode

## BREATHING EXPERIMENT

Place your right hand on your belly and your left hand on your chest and take a deep breath in. Notice which hand rises first and if your shoulders shrug upwards. If your left hand moves first then, like most of us, you are a chest breather. This has become a natural breathing pattern for most of us because of our slumped posture or desire to have a flat belly, but it is far from optimal. When we chest breathe, instead of using our diaphragm we are relying on the accessory chest muscles, which will limit our oxygen supply and leave us with tense shoulders and a stressed mindset.

If you look at a child breathing you will see their belly rise as they inhale and fall as they exhale. They are belly breathers. By using the diaphragm and pushing the belly out as we inhale we increase our lung capacity and allow more oxygen to flow into our bodies.

Aim to belly breathe whenever you can, especially at times of stress or when you want to relax during yin poses. There are several breathing exercises on the next few pages that you can perform before, during or after your Yoga Gym workout or at various times throughout the day to enhance your overall well-being.

# Ocean Breath

This is a form of breathing you can do before you work out and use throughout your training or yoga session to help you focus. Traditionally called 'Ujjayi', I call it Ocean Breath here because the noise you make is similar to the sound you hear when you hold a seashell up to your ear. It expands the lungs by dynamically pulling fresh air into them and expelling stale air.

**1.** Sit or stand comfortably with your spine upright and take a couple of long deep breaths.

**2.** Inhale through your nose, and exhale through your mouth. With each exhalation make a 'hhhaaaaa' sound as if you are trying to steam up a mirror.

**3.** Now continue to make the same sound as you exhale, but close your mouth so you are constricting the back of your throat to make a soft ocean sound (you may also sound like Darth Vadar!).

TIPS

Use Ocean Breath at the beginning of your workout or yoga practice to help heat the body.

If you come across a stressful situation in life then use Ocean Breath to keep calm.

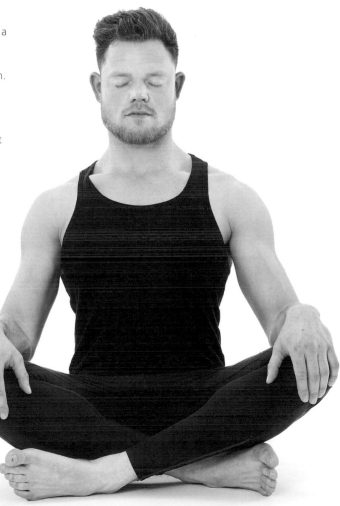

# Yang poses

**Yang poses are challenging and dynamic. They create length and strength in the muscles using the power of your own bodyweight. The challenging nature of these poses forces you to use all muscles from the centre of your core to the tips of your toes.**

Traditional strength training using weights relies heavily on concentric muscle contraction, which means the muscle gets shortened as it contracts. This can lead to permanently short, tight muscles. Yang poses, however, use a combination of eccentric muscle contraction, whereby the muscle lengthens when under tension, and isometric muscle contraction, whereby the muscle does not change length, so you can get strong without compromising suppleness.

The strength gains you will achieve through yang poses will be matched by increases in flexibility. As you contract muscles on one side of a joint to build strength, you automatically stretch the muscles on the opposite side of the joint to develop suppleness. For example, when you straighten your leg by contracting the muscles at the front of your thigh (quadriceps) you stretch the muscles at the back of your thigh (hamstrings). The more powerfully you can contract your quadriceps, the more your hamstrings will relax and the better the stretch you will feel.

## BENEFITS OF YANG POSES

Yang poses develop muscular strength and endurance through eccentric and isometric contraction, improving core strength and building muscle size to create a toned body. Focusing upon and isolating key muscles teaches body awareness and stimulates the flow of energy around the body, and by lengthening muscles at the same time as strengthening them, flexibility is improved.

## HOW TO PERFORM YANG POSES

- Perform the Stabilising Sequence (see p. 48) before moving into the pose.
- Hold each pose for 5–10 breaths.
- Take the basic form of the pose then refine it by contracting and relaxing specific muscles.
- Lengthen your spine and lift your chest as you inhale. Relax and release or twist deeper into the pose as you exhale.
- Keep a long spine throughout the pose.
- Create stability in the pose by co-contracting (simultaneously contracting two or more muscles) all the muscles either side of the joint.

# Mountain

**TARGET AREAS**

**Strengthens:** Full body
**Hold Time:** 5–10 breaths

Mastering your posture is the first step in building functional strength and improving flexibility. Mountain pose literally teaches us how to stand on our own two feet (which is harder than you think if you sit at a desk all day!). By bringing consciousness to your posture, Mountain pose realigns the spine, stabilises the core and brings the body back into balance.

**1.** Bring your feet, ankles and knees together and straighten your legs.

**2.** Use the Stabilising Sequence (see p. 48) to align your spine.

**3.** Straighten your arms either side of your body with your palms facing forwards or bring your palms into Prayer Hands (see p. 48) in front of your chest.

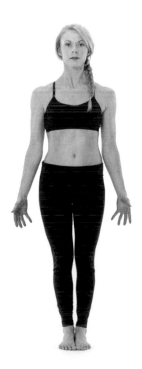
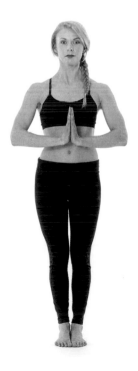

**TIPS**

Use Mountain pose to check in with your body before and after each standing pose to assess how your body feels.

There is a reciprocal relationship between how you stand and how you feel. When you feel tired or anxious this is reflected in a slumped and defeated posture. When you stand tall in Mountain pose you create confidence and openness.

Try Mountain pose when you're in supermarket queues, on the phone, waiting for a train, or anytime when you find yourself standing around.

# Twisted Chair

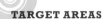

**Strengthens:** Core, thighs, bottom, lower back, ankles and calves
**Stretches:** Waist, shoulders and upper back
**Hold Time:** 5–10 breaths each side

**As well as whittling your waist and toning your thighs, Twisted Chair helps to cleanse the body. Twists squeeze out toxins from your internal organs to improve digestion and circulation.**

**1.** Begin in Chair Pose (see p. 62) with your hands in Prayer Hands position (see p. 50) in front of your chest. On an exhalation, bring your right elbow across your body to the outside of your left knee.

**2.** Press your palms firmly together and aim to bring your breastbone up to meet your thumbs. Check that your knees are together and that one of your knees is not falling forwards, then look up to the sky.

**3.** To exit the pose, twist back to centre and repeat on the other side, resting in between if you need to.

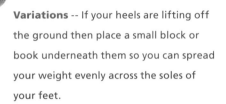

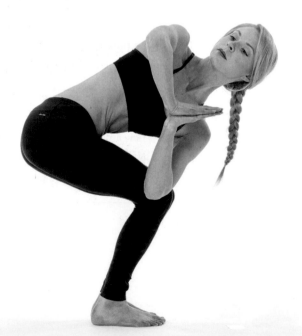

**Variations** -- If your heels are lifting off the ground then place a small block or book underneath them so you can spread your weight evenly across the soles of your feet.

**Take it up a notch** -- To deepen the pose, spread your arms wide once you have twisted, with your top fingertips reaching towards the sky and your bottom fingertips stretching towards the floor.

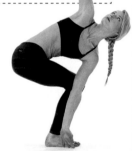

**TIPS**

Aim to rotate from your core, allowing your chest, shoulders and head to follow.

Draw your shoulder blades together to help deepen the twist and open your chest to the sky.

# Standing Forward Bend

## TARGET AREAS

**Strengthens:** Back, core and quadriceps
**Stretches:** Hamstrings, calves and back
**Hold Time:** 5–10 breaths

**TIPS**

Pulling up on your kneecaps and engaging the front of your thighs will help to release your hamstrings.

Play around with shifting your weight between the heels and balls of your feet and notice how the stretch changes.

**Being able to touch our toes is something we do very naturally as kids but many adults struggle with it. The focus in a Standing Forward Bend is to use the strength of the lower back and core to keep the spine long so you get a strong stretch in the back of your legs.**

**1.** Begin with your feet about hip-width apart. Squeeze your bottom, brace your belly and bring your hands to your hips.

**2.** As you exhale, hinge forwards from your hips, keeping your spine long. Bring your hands down to take hold of your big toes with your two forefingers. With each inhalation lift and lengthen your spine by looking ahead of you, and with each exhalation, pull yourself deeper into the pose using the strength of your biceps.

**3.** To exit the pose, lift and lengthen as you inhale, bring your hands to your hips as you exhale, and come back to standing on your next inhalation.

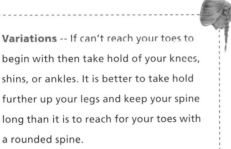

**Variations** -- If can't reach your toes to begin with then take hold of your knees, shins, or ankles. It is better to take hold further up your legs and keep your spine long than it is to reach for your toes with a rounded spine.

**Take it up a notch** -- If you can reach your toes easily then bring your hands beneath your feet so you are standing on your palms, aiming to get your toes up to your wrist joints.

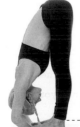

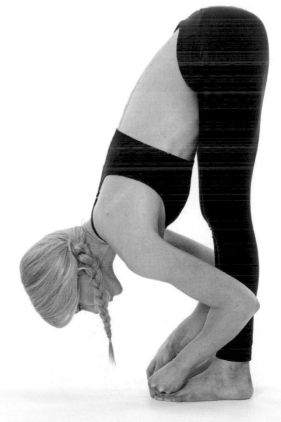

# Head to Knee

TARGET AREAS

**Strengthens:** Core and ankles
**Stretches:** Hamstrings, bottom, calves
and shoulders
**Hold Time:** 5–10 breaths

**This pose focuses on stretching the hamstring and calf of the front leg. By having your hands in Reverse Prayer (see p. 192), Head to Knee pose also stretches the shoulders, showing how yoga works the body as a synergistic unit rather than just isolating individual muscles.**

**1.** Begin in Mountain pose (see p. 59) and take a step back with your right leg so that your feet are about 1m (3ft 4in) apart. Keep the toes of your left foot facing forwards and turn your right foot out by 45 degrees.

**2.** Bring your hands into Reverse Prayer, pushing your palms together and pulling your elbows back. On an exhalation, soften your right knee slightly and fold forwards as if you are bringing your chin to your shin. Straighten your left leg and push your right hip forwards to keep your hips parallel. Lift and lengthen with each inhalation and release deeper with each exhalation.

**3.** To exit the pose, bend your front knee and push back to standing on an inhalation. Step your feet together and repeat with your right foot forwards.

**Variations** -- If you have very tight shoulders then rest your fingers on the floor instead of putting your hands in Reverse Prayer.

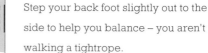

**TIPS**

Step your back foot slightly out to the side to help you balance – you aren't walking a tightrope.

**Lift your elbows to the sky to help keep your spine long.**

# Standing Wide Leg Forward Bend

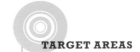

**TARGET AREAS**

**Strengthens:** Ankles and quadriceps
**Stretches:** Inner thighs, hamstrings and calves
**Hold Time:** 5–10 breaths

**TIPS**

Push your weight into the outside edge of your feet to ease any pressure on your ankle.

If you want a pose that will help to relieve tightness in your inner thighs then this is for you. It is also an **inversion** in that your head is below your heart so it will help to shift your nervous system from fight-or-flight mode to resting and digesting.

**1.** Begin in a wide stance and spread your arms out to the side, parallel to the floor. Position your ankles underneath your wrists and keep your feet parallel with your toes facing forwards. Bring your hands to your hips and, as you inhale, lengthen your spine. As you exhale, fold forwards by hinging at your hips.

**2.** Bring your hands down to the floor shoulder-width apart so that your fingertips are in line with your toes. With each inhalation, lengthen your spine and look forwards and with each exhalation draw yourself deeper into the pose by bending your arms.

**3.** To exit the pose, soften your knees, return your hands to your hips and come back to standing on an inhalation.

> **Variations** -- Play around with hand placements by keeping your hands on your hips, taking hold of your toes, or interlocking your fingers behind your back and bringing your hands up and over your head as you fold forwards.

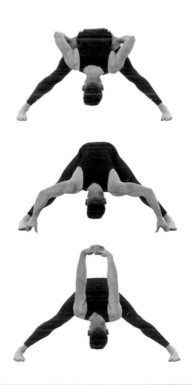

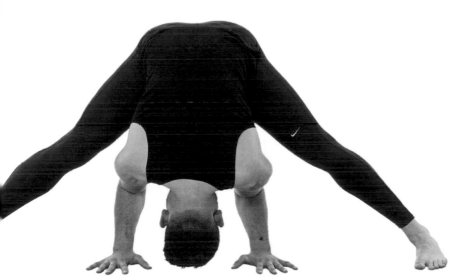

# Side Angle

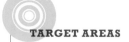

**TARGET AREAS**

**Strengthens:** Thighs and hip flexors (the group of muscles at the front of the hip)
**Stretches:** Inner thighs and waist
**Hold Time:** 5–10 breaths each side

This pose will help to build strength in the thighs at the same time as stretching the groin. Side Angle is the perfect pose during which to use your Ocean Breath (see p. 53) in. By opening your chest, the pose allows you to deepen your inhalations and relax into the exhalations.

**1.** Begin in a wide stance with your toes facing forwards, then turn your left foot in about 30 degrees and your right foot out 90 degrees. Spread your arms so they are parallel to the floor and use the Stabilising Sequence (see p. 48) to stabilise your pelvis. As you exhale, bend your right knee, bring your right fingertips to the floor inside your right foot, and send your left arm up and over your head as if you are throwing a spear.

**2.** As you flex your torso over your front thigh, rotate your chest upwards from your belly so you are looking up and under your left armpit. Focus on dropping your hips so your front thigh is parallel to the floor, simultaneously extending through the tips of your fingers.

**3.** Exit the pose on an inhalation by pushing back to centre, straightening the front leg and reversing your feet. Repeat on the other side.

**TIPS**

Aim to create one diagonal line of energy from the outside of your back foot up through the fingertips of your top hand.

If your front knee is falling inwards then use your front elbow to pin it back.

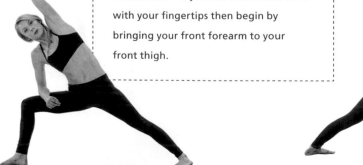

**Variations** -- If you can't reach the floor with your fingertips then begin by bringing your front forearm to your front thigh.

**Take it up a notch** -- If you want more of a stretch, drop your top arm behind your back and bring your bottom arm underneath your front thigh. Attempt to interlock your fingers to bind the pose by sinking your hips and rotating your chest to the sky.

# Twisted Side Angle

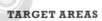

## TARGET AREAS

**Strengthens:** Thighs, hip flexors and core

**Stretches:** Hips, bottom and back

**Hold Time:** 5–10 breaths

**TIPS**

Aim to bring your sternum up to meet your thumbs at the same time as pushing your palms together.

**Push your weight through your back foot to help you balance.**

Twisted Side Angle works your lower body and your core. The shoulders turn in one direction and the hips rotate in the opposite direction using the power of your core to produce a detoxifying twist.

**1.** Begin in Mountain pose (see p. 59) and step your left foot back about 1.5m (5ft), keeping your heels in line. Drop your left knee to the floor and press your left elbow against the outside of your right knee to turn your torso.

**2.** Bring your right hand to meet your left hand in Prayer Hands (see p. 50) and use your core strength to twist your upper body towards your right leg. Lift your left knee off the floor and straighten the leg. Focus on squeezing your torso against your front thigh without letting your thigh drift inwards.

**3.** To exit the pose, drop your left knee to the floor, release the twist and return to Mountain pose before repeating on the other leg.

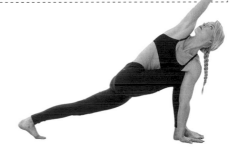

**Variations** -- If you're struggling to straighten the back leg, then do it with your knee on the floor until you have built the strength in your quadriceps and buttocks.

**Take it up a notch** -- To make the pose more challenging, place your lower hand on the floor to the outside of the front foot and lengthen your top hand to the sky.

# Warrior 3

**Strengthens:** Thighs, hip flexors, bottom, lower back and shoulders
**Stretches:** Bottom, hamstrings and calves
**Hold Time:** 5–10 breaths

**TIPS**

If you feel you are losing your balance, then bend your standing leg slightly to lower your centre of gravity.

**Warrior 3 is a balancing act that improves strength through your core. Building a stable foundation prevents your arms and legs wavering so you can refine the pose to get a better stretch in the hamstring of the standing leg.**

**1.** Begin in Warrior 1 (see p. 72) with your right foot forwards. Launch forwards, lifting your left leg until both your torso and rear leg are parallel to the floor. Find something stable in front of you to focus on.

**2.** Squeeze your right buttock and pull up on your right kneecap to stabilise the standing leg, focusing on keeping both hips level. Pull your shoulders away from your ears to engage your upper back muscles and keep your spine long.

**3.** To exit the pose, soften your left leg and relax into Mountain pose (see p. 59) before repeating on the other side.

**Variations** -- Begin with the toes of your rear leg on the floor, lifting it higher as you gain strength and suppleness.

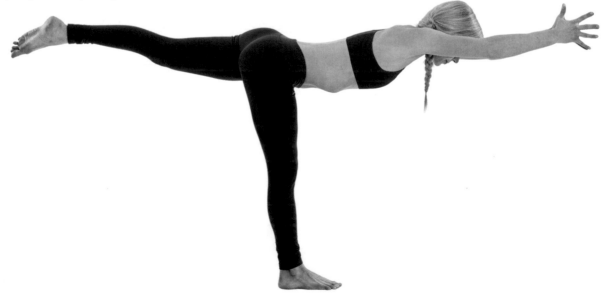

# Reverse Warrior

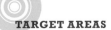

**TARGET AREAS**

**Strengthens:** Thighs and shoulders
**Stretches:** Hips, hamstrings, inner thighs and waist
**Hold Time:** 5–10 breaths

Sink your hips deeper with each exhalation.

Make sure your front knee does not fall inwards. Aim to keep it in line with the ankle.

**Reverse Warrior is great for stretching and strengthening the body. The pose builds strength in the front thigh at the same time as opening the chest and stretching the entire upper body, which will lengthen the spine and leave you feeling confident and determined.**

**1.** Begin in Warrior 2 (see p. 73) with your left leg bent. Lean back so that your right hand reaches down your right hamstring and your left-hand fingertips point towards the sky with your palm facing backwards.

**2.** Focus on keeping your hips open and your front thigh parallel to the floor at the same time as lifting your chest towards the sky so you feel a stretch in your waist.

**3.** Come out of the pose by returning to Warrior 2 on an inhalation. Repeat on the other leg.

**Take it up a notch** -- To increase the stretch in your shoulders, bring your arms into Cow Face Arms (see p. 191) by dropping your top hand behind your head and bringing the hand reaching down the rear leg up behind your back to clasp the fingers.

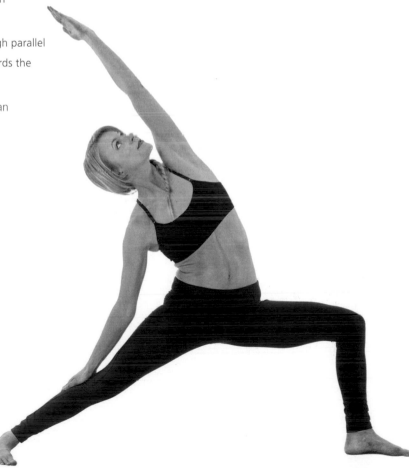

# Tree Pose

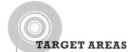

**Strengthens:** Core, thighs, hip flexors, back and shoulders
**Stretches:** Hips and inner thighs
**Hold Time:** 5–10 breaths each side

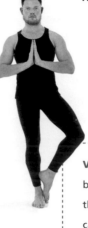

**Tree pose builds stability and flexibility. Remember to root yourself firmly to the ground through your standing foot to help you balance and keep your core and back muscles strong to provide stability. The more stable you feel, the more you will be able to open the hip of the bent leg and experience both the strengthening and lengthening benefits of the pose.**

**1.** Begin in Mountain pose (see p. 59) and bring your left foot up to your inner thigh, using your hands to lift the foot if necessary. Bring your hands into Prayer Hands (see p. 50) in front of your chest.

**2.** Squeeze your buttocks to stabilise the standing leg and deepen the stretch in the hip of your bent leg by consciously drawing your knee backwards.

**3.** Return to Mountain pose before repeating on the other leg.

**Variations** -- If your hips feel tight then begin with your toes on the floor or with the sole of your foot resting against your calf. Try to avoid resting on the inner knee as this puts pressure on the joint.

**Take it up a notch** -- To deepen the pose, bring the heel of the bent leg into the hip crease of the opposite leg with your knee pointing towards the floor.

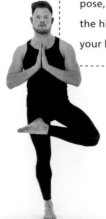

**TIPS**

Spread your weight evenly between all four corners of your standing foot to help you balance.

# Eagle Pose

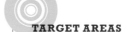

**TARGET AREAS**

**Strengthens:** Core, thighs, hip flexors and chest
**Stretches:** Shoulders and bottom
**Hold Time:** 5–10 breaths each side

**TIPS**

Find something still in front of you to focus on, to help you balance.

**Don't be put off by the pretzel-like positioning of the arms and legs, as Eagle Pose is a great stretch for the back of the shoulders and buttocks and builds strength in the thighs – all done standing on one leg! Unlike other standing postures, which lift the chest, Eagle Pose folds the body forwards to draw energy inwards.**

**1.** Begin in Mountain pose (see p. 59) and bring your arms into Eagle Arms by crossing your left arm over your right, bending your elbows so your forearms are vertical and then bringing your palms together. Next, bend your knees and cross your right leg over your left, squeeze your thighs together and hook the toes of your right foot behind your left calf.

**2.** Drop your hips, lift your elbows and wrap your shoulder blades around the back of your ribcage to stretch your upper back,

**3.** To exit the pose, unravel your arms and your legs and return to Mountain pose. Repeat on the opposite side.

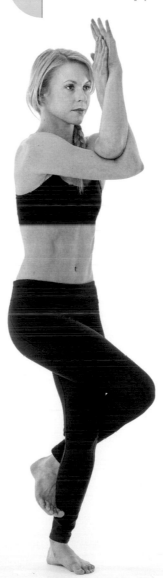

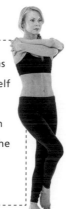

**Variations --** If you can't get your palms together in Eagle Arms then give yourself a hug by wrapping your arms around yourself. And If your hips feel tight then cross your knees, leaving your toes on the floor on the outside of your standing foot to help you balance.

# Table Top

**TARGET AREAS**

**Strengthens:** Core and shoulders

**TIPS**

Look at yourself from the side in a mirror to see if your back is flat.

**Like Mountain pose (see p. 59), the focus of Table Top is to ensure the spine is stable. We use Table Top as a way to get into other postures such as Bear (see p. 79) and Down Dog (see p. 80) and also as a position of rest.**

**1.** Come on to your hands and knees with your hands positioned directly below your shoulders and your knees positioned below your hips.

**2.** Use the Stabilising Sequence (see p. 48) by squeezing your bottom, bracing your belly, and drawing your shoulders away from your ears and down your back. Look at the floor just in front of you to keep your spine neutral.

**3.** Engage your pelvic floor and use your abdominal lock by drawing your belly button to your spine and your abdomen up and into your ribcage to stabilise the core.

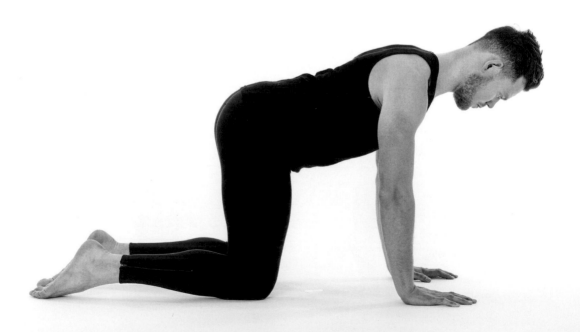

# Bear

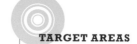

**TARGET AREAS**

**Strengthens:** Core, shoulders, and thighs
**Stretches:** Upper back
**Hold Time:** 5–10 breaths

**This is a great pose to build strength and stamina in the thighs and activate the core.**

**1.** Begin in Table Top (see p. 78), hook your toes under and lift your kneecaps off the floor so they are hovering about 20cm (8in) off the ground.

**2.** Focus on keeping your spine in a straight line with just its natural S-curve.

**3.** Release your knees to the mat on an exhalation.

**TIPS**

Dig your fingertips into the floor to activate the muscles in your forearms and ease any pressure on the wrists.

Look at the floor just in front of you to keep you neck in alignment with the rest of your spine.

**Take it up a notch** -- Make your core work harder by doing Three-legged Bear. Lift one foot off the ground, keeping your core strong and hips even.

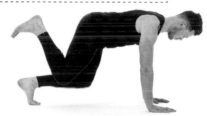

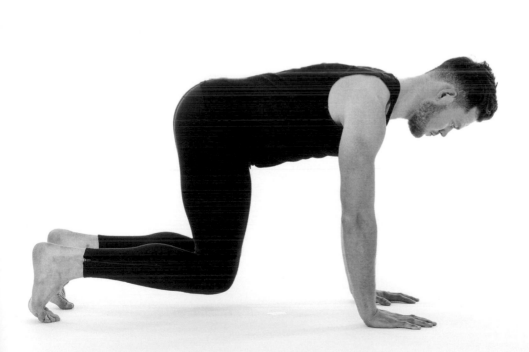

# Down Dog

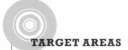

**Strengthens:** Thighs, hip flexors, shoulders and wrists
**Stretches:** Hamstrings, calves and back
**Hold Time:** 5–10 breaths

**TIPS**

Focus on pushing your bottom to the sky as you inhale and releasing your heels closer to the floor as you exhale.

Spread your fingers wide and push the floor away from you through your fingertips to reduce pressure on the wrists.

Down Dog is one of the most popular poses because it strengthens and stretches the body as well as acting as a physical barometer for how your body feels in between other poses and flows. It is a key part of the Sun Salutations (see p. 116) and shows how each part of your body works in harmony with the other parts – the looser your hamstrings are, the less pressure you will feel on your shoulders.

**1.** Begin in Table Top (see p. 78) and hook your toes under. Slowly straighten your legs to push your bottom to the sky so you are in an upturned V-shape. Check your hands are shoulder-width apart and your feet are hip-width apart.

**2.** Refine the pose by making sure your arms are straight, pulling up your kneecaps to engage the front of your thighs, and looking back between your legs.

**3.** Exit the pose by bending your knees to the mat to return to Table Top.

**Variations** -- If the backs of your legs are feeling particularly tight then spread your feet wider or walk your Dog by bending your knees one at a time.

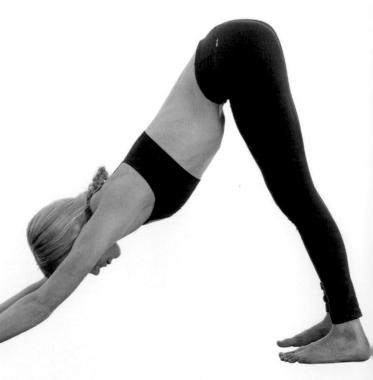

# Three-legged Dog

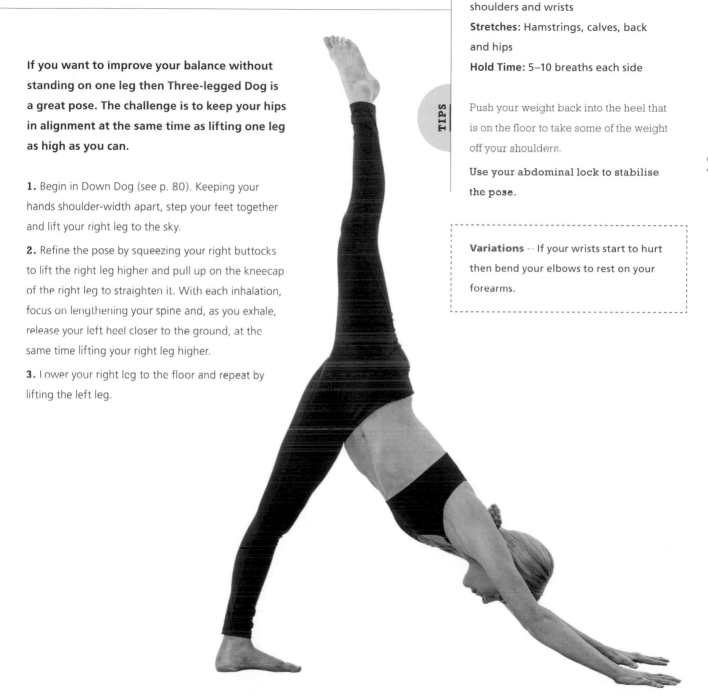

**If you want to improve your balance without standing on one leg then Three-legged Dog is a great pose. The challenge is to keep your hips in alignment at the same time as lifting one leg as high as you can.**

**1.** Begin in Down Dog (see p. 80). Keeping your hands shoulder-width apart, step your feet together and lift your right leg to the sky.

**2.** Refine the pose by squeezing your right buttocks to lift the right leg higher and pull up on the kneecap of the right leg to straighten it. With each inhalation, focus on lengthening your spine and, as you exhale, release your left heel closer to the ground, at the same time lifting your right leg higher.

**3.** Lower your right leg to the floor and repeat by lifting the left leg.

**TARGET AREAS**

**Strengthens:** Thighs, hips flexors, shoulders and wrists
**Stretches:** Hamstrings, calves, back and hips
**Hold Time:** 5–10 breaths each side

**TIPS**

Push your weight back into the heel that is on the floor to take some of the weight off your shoulders.

**Use your abdominal lock to stabilise the pose.**

**Variations** -- If your wrists start to hurt then bend your elbows to rest on your forearms.

# Dolphin

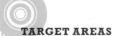
**TARGET AREAS**

**Strengthens:** Thighs, hip flexors and shoulders
**Stretches:** Hamstrings, calves, back and shoulders
**Hold Time:** 5–10 breaths

**TIPS**

The more forcefully you can root yourself into the ground the easier you will find it to lift your shoulders and hips away from the base of the pose.

**Let your head hang freely so there is no tension in your neck.**

**Dolphin is a great alternative to Down Dog (see p. 80) if you have any wrist issues. It is also brilliant for opening and strengthening the upper body and helping you get used to being upside down, and as a way in to more challenging poses such as Forearm Stand (see p. 194).**

**1.** Begin in Table Top (see p. 78) and bend your elbows to bring your forearms to the ground with your palms facing down. Hook your toes under and straighten your legs in the same way you would in Down Dog. Aim to keep your forearms parallel and look back between your legs.

**2.** Press your forearms into the ground and lift your shoulders and hips away from the floor. Press your chest back towards your thighs and release your heels closer to the ground with each exhalation.

**3.** To exit the pose, bend your knees to the ground and straighten your arms to return to Table Top.

**Variations** -- If your shoulders are too tight for you to be able to keep your forearms parallel, allow your hands to come together so your forearms form a triangle and bring your palms together in Prayer Hands (see p. 50).

**Take it up a notch** -- Bring your feet together and lift one leg to the sky to challenge your balance.

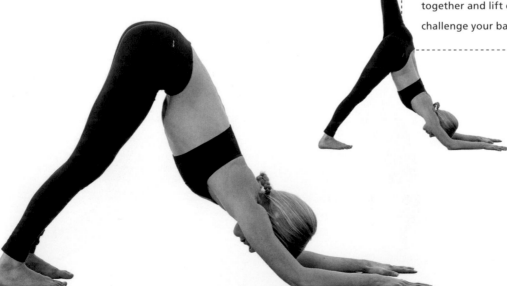

# Crouching Tiger

**TARGET AREAS**

**Strengthens:** Core, shoulders, wrists and legs

**Hold Time:** 5–10 breaths

**TIPS**

Imagine you are about to jump up to Handstand (see p. 194) from this position to really activate the backs of your legs.

**Crouching Tiger is the position you get into before you jump your feet from Down Dog (see p. 80) in between your hands in the Sun Salutations (see p. 116). Really focus on engaging your core in this pose, strengthening your shoulders and tightening your hamstrings so you can get as much power as possible.**

**1.** Begin in Down Dog, come up on to your toes, bend your knees very slightly and look between your hands.

**2.** Once you have taken the basic form of the pose, refine it by engaging your core and lifting your bottom to the sky to activate your hamstrings.

**3.** Exit the pose by straightening your legs and returning to Down Dog, or by jumping your feet between your hands.

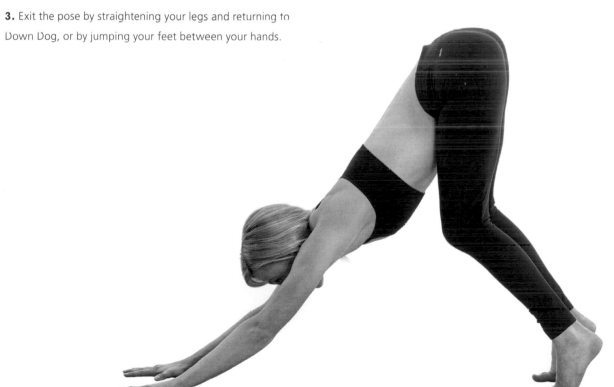

# Planche Plank

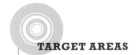
**Strengthens:** Core, shoulders, bottom, upper arms and wrists

**Hold Time:** 5–10 breaths

**This pose builds core and shoulder strength and puts your body in the perfect position to tackle arm balances such as Crow (see p. 87).**

**1.** Begin in Plank (see p. 84) and shift your weight forwards so that your shoulders are about 50cm (20in) in front of your wrists.

**2.** Stabilise the pose by keeping your core tight and drawing your shoulders away from your ears to keep your neck long. Look slightly in front of you to keep your spine in alignment.

**3.** To come out of the pose, shift your shoulders back over your wrists and release to Table Top (see p. 78).

**Variations** -- To make the pose less challenging, place your hands on a raised surface such as a stall, a yoga block or a pile of books.

**Take it up a notch** -- You can make this pose more challenging by raising your feet on a yoga block or chair.

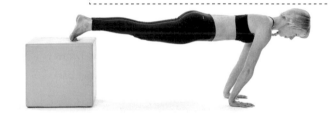

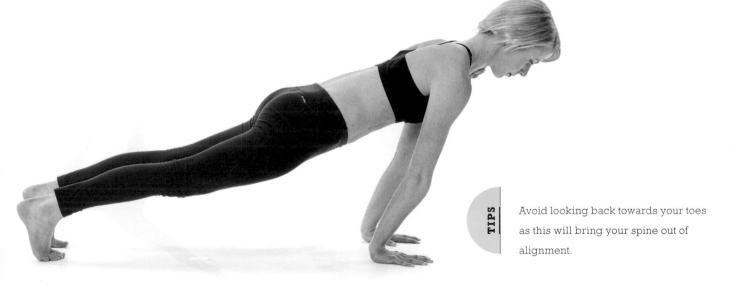

**TIPS**

Avoid looking back towards your toes as this will bring your spine out of alignment.

# Crow

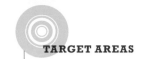

**TARGET AREAS**

**Strengthens:** Core, shoulders and wrists
**Stretches:** Upper back and hamstrings
**Hold Time:** 5–10 breaths

**TIPS**

Although this is an arm balance, a lot of the strength comes from the core. Focus on engaging your abdominals to release some of the pressure from your shoulders.

Arm balances require a combination of strength, balance and focus. Grounding yourself through your hands to provide a stable foundation is essential for giving you the confidence to lift your feet off the floor. The stronger your core is the less weight your knees will place on your upper arms and the longer you will be able to float in Crow.

**1.** Begin in Mountain pose (see p. 59) and squat down to the floor, coming up on to your toes if you can't keep your heels down. Spread your feet so they are slightly wider than hip-width apart and place your hands on the floor in front of you shoulder-width apart. Lift your bottom by straightening your legs just enough so that when you lean forwards and bring your shoulders in front of your wrists you can snuggle your knees into your armpits. Slowly transfer the weight into your hands, lift your toes off the ground and bring your heels together.

**2.** Once you have found your balance, refine the pose by bringing your toes towards your tailbone so you are rounding your spine. Activate your abdominal muscles to lift your torso upwards and reduce the amount of pressure on your arms.

**3.** Rock slowly backwards on to your toes to exit the pose.

**Variations** -- If you find it difficult to get your knees into your armpits then you can keep your arms bent and rest your knees on your upper arms.

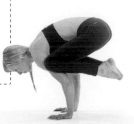

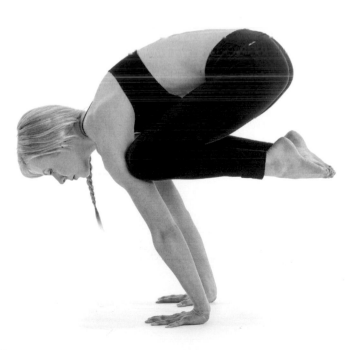

# Crocodile

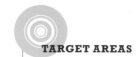

**Strengthens:** Core, shoulders, arms, chest, back and wrists

**Hold Time:** 5–10 breaths

**TIPS**

Engage the bottom and core muscles equally to stabilise the pelvis.

Think about pushing your lower back to the sky to activate your core and stop your pelvis sagging.

**If you struggle with push-ups then Crocodile pose will teach your body which muscles to engage in the bottom position. It is a key pose in the Sun Salutations (see p. 116) and is great to combine with Down Dog (see p. 80), Up Dog (see p. 102) and Plank (see p. 84) as well as being performed as a free-standing posture to build full body strength.**

**1.** Begin lying on your front with your palms on the floor either side of your chest and your elbows tucked in. Press your hands into the ground to lift your chest about 30cm (12in) off the floor. Hook your toes under, lift your knees off the floor by straightening your legs and lift your hips like a suspension bridge.

**2.** Once you are in position, stabilise the pose by squeezing your bottom and bracing your belly. Draw your shoulder blades towards the midline of your body and pull your shoulders away from your ears. Keep your core engaged to prevent your hips from sagging and attempt to scrub your hands forwards and toes backwards.

**3.** Slowly lower yourself down to the ground to exit the pose.

**Variations** -- Lifting your hips is challenging, so you can begin by placing a block underneath your pelvis to support your weight. You can also lower down from Plank to Crocodile, which can be easier then pushing up from the floor.

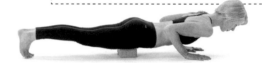

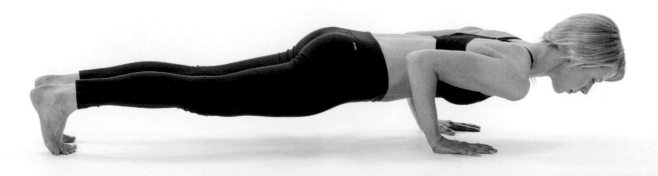

# Boat

**Boat pose builds stamina as well as strength. If you find it tough to activate your abdominal muscles then use this pose to learn how to brace your core.**

**1.** Begin seated with your knees bent and feet flat on the floor. Lean back as you lift your feet off the floor so the only thing in contact with the ground is your bottom. Straighten your legs so you are in a V-shape and bring your arms either side of your legs parallel to the floor.

**2.** Contract your abdominals and hip flexors so you can maintain the V-shape, pull up on your kneecaps to straighten your legs fully and squeeze your knees together. Arch your back slightly to prevent your spine from rounding and lift your chest forwards.

**3.** Release the pose by bending your legs and returning your feet to the floor with control.

**TARGET AREAS**

**Strengthens:** Core, hip flexors and upper back

**TIPS**

Notice how squeezing your knees together makes it easier to activate your abdominals.

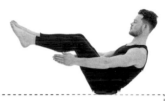

**Variations** -- If you find it tough to straighten your legs then keep your knees bent with your toes hovering just off the floor in Baby Boat. Hold on to the back of your thighs if you need to.

**Take it up a notch** -- Have a go at Boat with your arms above your head to challenge your core further.

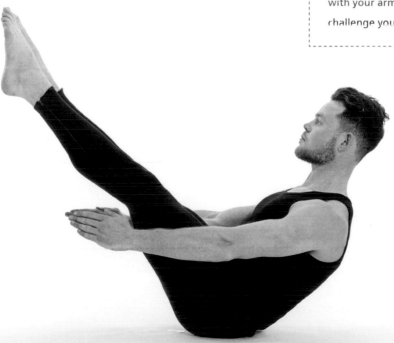

# Low Boat

**Strengthens:** Core
**Hold Time:** 5–10 breaths

**TIPS**

Squeeze your knees together to engage your abdominals more strongly.

Keep your breath strong to get as much oxygen to your muscles as possible.

**Low Boat builds strength in the core and helps to stabilise the spine. These are both essential when doing more challenging poses such as Handstand (see p. 194). Taking the time to master the basics such as core strength and spinal stability will pay off greatly as you further your yoga practice.**

**1.** Begin lying on your back with your legs lengthened out on the floor and your arms by your sides. Brace your belly and push your lower back towards the floor at the same time maintaining the natural curve of your spine, and slowly raise your shoulders and legs off the floor about 20cm (8in).

**2.** Focus on keeping your bottom squeezed and belly braced to prevent your lower back from over-arching.

**3.** Lower yourself back down to the ground, moving slowly and steadily.

**Take it up a notch** -- Make the pose more challenging by reaching your arms above your head.

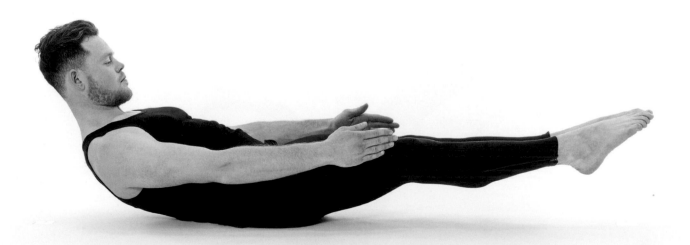

# Staff

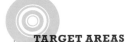

**TARGET AREAS**

**Strengthens:** Back, quadriceps and hip flexors

**Stretches:** Hamstrings and calves

**TIPS**

Imagine you have a string attached to the top of your head that is pulling you to the sky, to keep your spine long.

Keep your neck in line with the rest of your spine by pulling your head back slightly.

Staff pose is a seated version of Mountain pose (see p. 59). It is great to do in between other postures to bring your body back into balance and assess any changes you feel in your body or mind. Tight hamstrings and a weak core can cause you to slump forwards in this pose so building strength and flexibility will make it more comfortable.

**1.** Begin seated with your legs straight out in front of you. Place your hands either side of you with your fingertips facing outwards.

**2.** Squeeze your knees together and attempt to lift your heels off the floor to activate your hip flexors. Pull your feet back as if they are up against a wall and engage the muscles at the front of your thighs to straighten your legs. Slightly arch your back and draw your shoulder blades together to lift your chest.

**3.** Exit the pose by releasing any conscious effort.

**Variations** -- If you find you are slumping forwards then bend your knees to release tightness from your hamstrings and work towards straightening your legs.

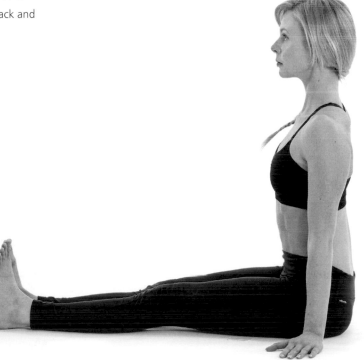

# Butterfly (yang)

**Strengthens:** Back and bottom
**Stretches:** Inner thighs
**Hold Time:** 5–10 breaths

**TIPS**

Open your feet as you would a book, so the soles of your feet are facing the ceiling. This will increase the external rotation of your hips to increase the stretch.

**We all have slight imbalances in our body, which may be anything from a slight curve of the spine to one hamstring that feels tighter than the other. Symmetrical poses such as Butterfly (yang) help to bring the body back into balance, specifically in the hips and the pelvis.**

**1.** Begin seated and bring the soles of your feet together. Take hold of your feet and pull your heels as close to your groin as possible.

**2.** Deepen the pose by squeezing your calves against your hamstrings to stabilise your knees. Squeeze your bottom to help open your hips and keep your spine long by drawing your shoulders down your back.

**3.** Exit the pose by bringing your hands to the outside of your thighs and drawing your knees together. Lengthen out your legs in front of you to rebalance the muscles you have stretched.

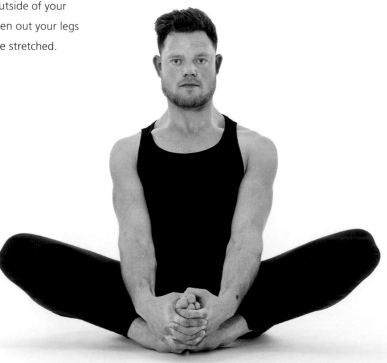

# Seated Wide Leg Forward Bend

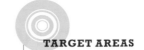

**TARGET AREAS**

**Strengthens:** Core and quadriceps
**Stretches:** Hamstrings, bottom, inner thighs and back
**Hold Time:** 5–10 breaths

**TIPS**

Keep the fronts of your thighs engaged to increase the stretch in your hamstrings.

Draw your shoulders down your back to prevent your spine from rounding.

Seated Wide Leg Forward Bend is a pose in which you can experience large physical and mental benefits through conscious refinement, rather than just hanging out in it passively.

**1.** Begin seated with your legs spread so they are open just wider than a right angle. Tilt the top of your pelvis forwards so you are sitting on the front of your sitting bones. Pull your feet back as if they are up against a wall and make sure that your kneecaps are pointing towards the ceiling. Inhale as you reach your hands to the sky, then as you exhale fold forwards by moving from the hip joint. Keep your arms above your head as long as possible, then when you can't hinge forwards any more bring your hands down to take hold of your shins, ankles, toes or the sides of your feet.

**2.** With each inhalation imagine your spine lengthening and as you exhale increase the forward bend by engaging the abdominals and the front of the thighs to draw you deeper into the pose.

**3.** Exit the pose on an inhalation, maintaining the length in your spine.

**Variations** -- Begin with bent legs if you need to or sit on a block or rolled-up blanket to make the pose more comfortable.

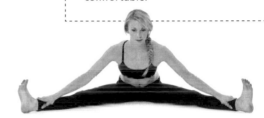

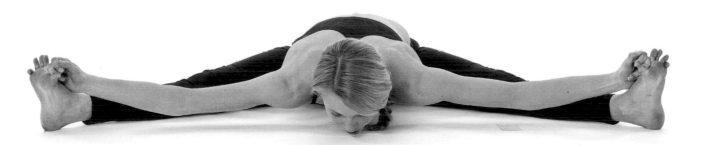

# Lotus

**Strengthens:** Hips, thighs and upper back
**Stretches:** Inner thighs and hips
**Hold Time:** 5–10 breaths each side

**TIPS**

Work up to this pose by performing other hip-opening postures and flows.

Keep a long spine by squeezing your bottom and bracing your belly.

**Lotus is a pose you automatically think of when it comes to yoga and it is also one of the most advanced hip-openers. You need to develop flexibility in the hips to prevent any pressure being placed on the knee in Lotus, so it is a good pose to build up to by performing other hip-openers such as Butterfly (yang) (see p. 94).**

**1.** Begin seated with your right leg crossed on top of your left leg. Take hold of your lower right leg and position your right heel into your left hip crease. Lift your left shin and place your left heel in your right hip crease.

**2.** Pull your toes back to activate the muscles in the backs of your legs and protect your knees. Squeeze your bottom and notice how this releases your knees closer to the ground.

**3.** Exit the pose by lifting your left leg off your right leg and releasing your right heel from your left hip crease. Lengthen your legs straight out in front of you, before repeating on the other side.

**Variations** -- Lotus is a strong hip-opener, so use Half Lotus to build up to it by bringing one heel into the opposite hip crease while leaving the other leg outstretched underneath.

**Take it up a notch** -- If Lotus feels comfortable then work your core in Floating Lotus by placing your hands either side of you and lifting your bottom off the floor.

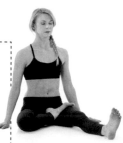

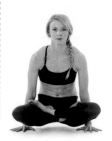

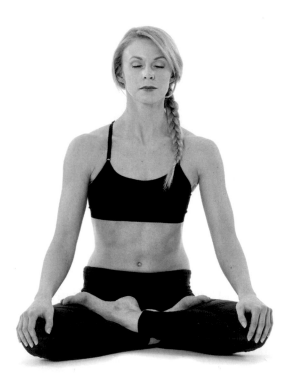

# Baby Cobra (yang)

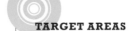

**TARGET AREAS**

**Strengthens:** Shoulders and back
**Hold Time:** 5–10 breaths

**TIPS**

Actively push the floor away through your forearms to strengthen your shoulders.

**Avoid collapsing your neck into your shoulders by drawing your shoulder blades together.**

**Baby Cobra (yang) is a gentle backbend that will nourish your spine and hips. If you sit hunched over a computer all day this is a great pose to reverse a slumped posture and open your chest.**

**1.** Begin by lying on your front with your arms bent and your palms on the floor just in front of your shoulders. Push your pubic bone into the floor and lift your chest by pressing your weight into your forearms.

**2.** Refine the pose by rolling your shoulders back and down and attempt to scrub your elbows backwards to open your chest forwards.

**3.** To exit the pose, slowly lower your chest back down to the floor and stretch out your arms.

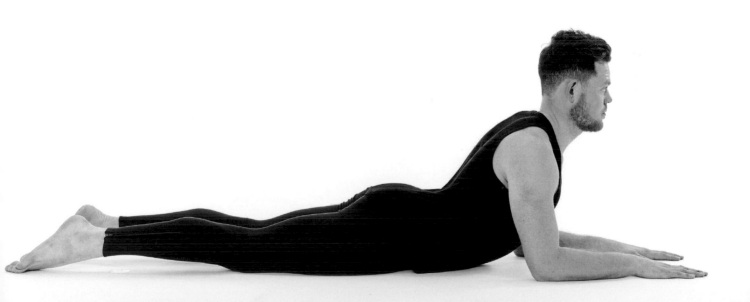

# Up Dog

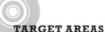
**Strengthens:** Shoulders, back, bottom, thighs and wrists
**Stretches:** Belly, chest and hip flexors
**Hold Time:** 5–10 breaths

**TIPS**

Press the mounds at the base of your index fingers into the floor to support your wrists.

**Focus the backbend on your upper back by lifting your heart centre forwards.**

**Up Dog is a great backbend that stretches the front of the body as well as strengthening the back of it. Taking the basic form of the pose and then refining it by focusing on each region will allow you to feel the full benefit and give your body an opportunity to learn the proper posture for when you use it in faster flows such as Sun Salutations (see p. 116).**

**1.** Begin lying on your front and bring your palms to rest either side of your chest. Slowly straighten your arms to lift your chest, straighten your legs and push the tops of your feet into the mat.

**2.** Refine the pose by rolling your shoulders back and away from your ears to open your chest. Engage the backs of your arms to keep your elbows straight and attempt to scrub your hands backwards. Keep the fronts of your thighs engaged by pulling up on your kneecaps and slightly firm your bottom to release any tightness in the fronts of your hips.

**3.** Release the pose by slowly lowering your chest back down to the ground or lifting your hips and rolling over your toes to Down Dog (see p. 80).

**Variations** -- If Up Dog is too challenging to begin with then remain in Baby Cobra (yang) (see p. 101).

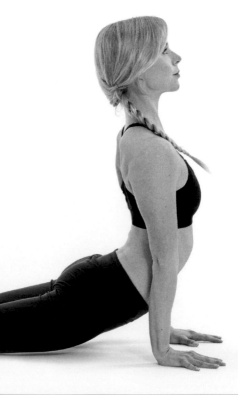

# Reverse Table Top

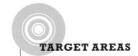

**TARGET AREAS**

**Strengthens:** Core, shoulders, bottom, upper arms and wrists

**Stretches:** Upper arms, belly, chest and thighs

**TIPS**

Push the floor away from you through your hands and feet to build a stable foundation.

Squeeze your bottom to help lift your hips.

**Reverse Table Top strengthens and stretches the entire body. Lifting your hips builds strength in the back of your body and tones your bottom and thighs. The stretch you feel in the front of the body in this pose shows you how contracting the muscles on one side of the body stretches out the muscles on the opposite side.**

**1.** Begin seated with your legs bent in front of you and the soles of your feet on the floor. Reach your hands back behind you with your fingertips facing forwards. Straighten your arms and draw your shoulder blades together to open the chest. Squeeze your bottom, lift your hips and let your head hang back.

**2.** Aim to align your knees over your ankles and your shoulders over your wrists. Keep your thighs parallel to help strengthen the inner thigh muscles.

**3.** Lower your hips down on an exhale and return to seated.

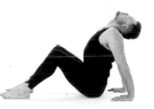

**Variations** -- If it is too challenging to lift your hips to begin with, then leave your bottom on the floor, reach your fingertips behind you, draw your shoulder blades together to open your chest and let your head hang back.

**Take it up a notch** -- You can make this pose more challenging by lifting one leg, pointing your toes to the sky.

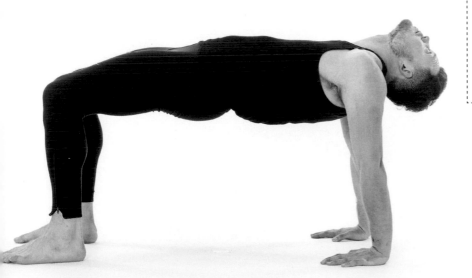

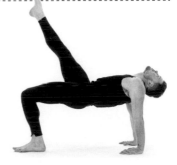

# Reverse Plank

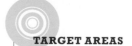
**Strengthens:** Core, shoulders, bottom, upper arms and wrists
**Stretches:** Upper arms, belly, chest and thighs
**Hold Time:** 5–10 breaths

**TIPS**

Draw your shoulder blades together to open your chest to the sky.

**Push the floor away through your hands to straighten your arms and stretch the front of your upper arms and your chest.**

**Reverse Plank stretches the front of the body as well as strengthening the entire back of the body. By letting your head fall back in this pose, you stretch the front of your neck and calm your mind.**

**1.** Begin seated with your legs bent in front of you with the soles of your feet on the floor. Lift your hips to Reverse Table Top (see p. 103) and walk your feet out in front of you to straighten your legs, keeping your toes on the ground. Allow your head to hang back.

**2.** Keep your bottom squeezed and arch your back to lift your hips up further. Pull up on your kneecaps, activate the front of your thighs and straighten your legs.

**3.** Ease out of the pose by bending your knees and elbows and lowering yourself to the floor.

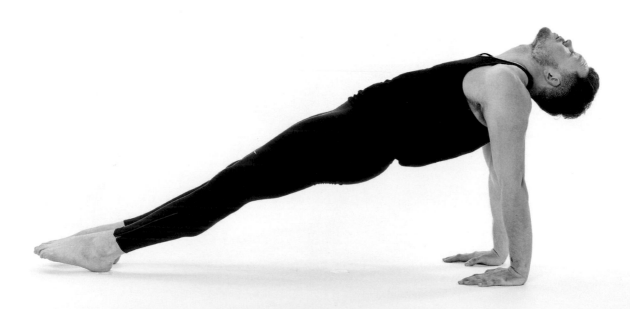

# Locust

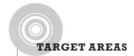

**Strengthens:** Back, bottom and thighs

**Hold Time:** 5–10 breaths

**TIPS**

Squeeze your knees together to help you engage your bottom and core.

Push your pubic bone into the floor to stabilise your pelvis.

**Locust pose is a baby backbend that requires flexibility, strength and muscular endurance. The pose brings awareness to which muscles are required to lift the chest and legs, building mind–muscle connections to enhance your practice.**

**1.** Begin lying on your belly with your arms by your sides and your palms facing towards your body. Squeeze your bottom and turn your big toes towards each other. As you exhale, lift your head, chest, arms and legs off the floor so you are resting on your hips and your belly.

**2.** Refine the pose by lengthening from the top of your head to your toes and lift your arms so they are parallel to the floor. Draw your shoulder blades together to lift your chest forwards and gaze at the floor ahead of you.

**3.** Release the pose by lowering your chest and legs slowly to the floor.

**Variations** -- Prepare for Locust using different variations of the pose. Focus on the upper body by interlacing your fingers behind your back and work on the lower body by leaving your chest on the floor and just lifting your legs.

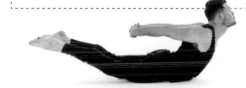

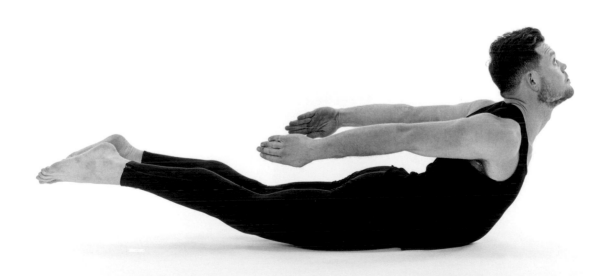

# Baby Bridge

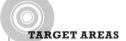

**Strengthens:** Back, bottom and hamstrings

**Stretches:** Shoulders, chest and hips

**TIPS**

Draw your chest towards your chin to increase the arch in your back.

Aim to keep your thighs parallel, which will help you engage your core and lift your hips.

**Baby Bridge works the entire body to build both strength and flexibility. Lifting your hips in this pose activates the muscles at the front of the thighs and the bottom to tone these areas, restore optimal spinal mobility, and stretch the belly and chest.**

**1.** Begin lying on your back with your knees bent and your feet flat on the floor, about hip-width apart. Squeeze your bottom and brace your belly so you are tipping the top of your pelvis backwards. Push your weight into your heels and lift your hips.

**2.** Lift your hips as high as you can using the strength of your buttocks, then activate your hamstrings by pushing your weight into your heels. Draw your shoulder blades together beneath you to lift your chest towards the sky and increase the stretch down the front of your body.

**3.** Exit the pose by slowly lowering back down to the ground one vertebrae at a time.

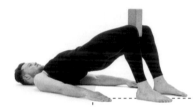

**Variations** -- Place a block between your knees to keep your thighs parallel and to help you to engage your core.

**Take it up a notch** -- Lift one leg to make the pose more challenging and add a stretch to your hamstring.

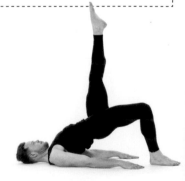

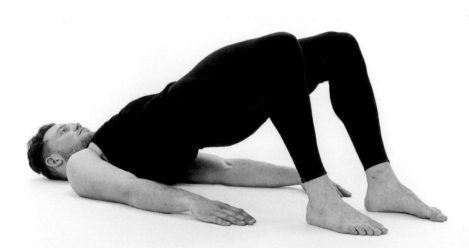

# Bridge

Also known as Wheel and Upward Bow pose, this is a deep backbend that relies on stability and flexibility. As a child you probably found going up into a Bridge a simple and fun thing to do, but after years or slumping at desks or sitting in cars all day, the body forgets how to move naturally and the mind becomes scared of trying new things. Be patient as you build up to Bridge in order to give your body time to strengthen and open.

**1.** Begin lying on your back with your knees bent, about hip-width apart. Place your hands just above your shoulders with your palms facing down and your forearms vertical. Without letting your elbows wing out, lift your hips, press your hands into the ground and straighten your arms to arch your back and lift your head off the floor.

**2.** Once you feel stable in the pose refine it by slightly firming your buttocks and engaging your quadriceps to straighten your knees. Externally rotate your shoulders to stabilise your upper body and draw your shoulder blades together.

**3.** To exit the pose, bend your elbows and walk your feet away from your bottom as you lower yourself down slowly to the ground.

**TARGET AREAS**

**Strengthens:** Back, bottom, hamstrings and shoulders
**Stretches:** Hips and quadriceps
**Hold Time:** 5–10 breaths

**TIPS**

To externally rotate your shoulders, imagine trying to rotate your hands outwards as they are stuck to the floor.

Deepen the pose by fixing your hands to the floor and attempting to scrub your hands towards your feet.

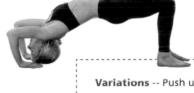

**Variations** -- Push up on to the top of your head if you haven't built the strength to straighten your arms.

**Take it up a notch** -- Lift one leg to make the pose more challenging and add a stretch to your hamstring.

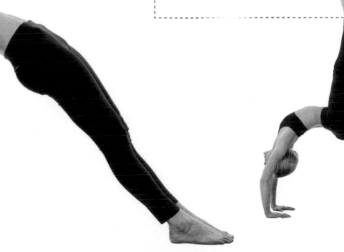

# Camel

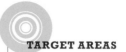
**Strengthens:** Bottom, upper back, core and hamstrings
**Stretches:** Spine, hip flexors, quadriceps, chest and shoulders
**Hold Time:** 5–10 breaths

**TIPS**

Keep your bottom firm throughout the pose to increase the stretch in the front of your hips and thighs.

**Press the tops of your feet into the floor to lift your pelvis.**

**Camel is a deep backbend that strengthens the entire back of the body as well as stretching the front of it. Leaning back and letting your head fall can seem scary to begin with, so start with the variations and work up to the full posture. The stronger your core is, the more stable you feel.**

**1.** Begin kneeling with your knees about hip-width apart. Place your hands on your lower back with your fingertips pointing down towards the floor. Squeeze your bottom and brace your belly to stabilise your pelvis. Draw your elbows towards each other to lift your chest to the sky and begin to arch backwards until you can place the palms of your hands on the soles of your feet.

**2.** Make sure your hips stay over your knees rather than drifting backwards by pressing the top of your feet into the floor to activate the fronts of the thighs. Gently engage your abdominals to protect the lower back and lift the pelvis.

**3.** Exit the pose slowly by bringing your hands to your lower back and returning your spine to neutral. Be careful not to rotate your spine on the way back to kneeling.

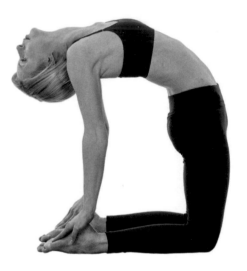

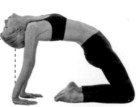

**Variations** -- Camel is a deep back bend so condition your body to get used to the movement with Baby Camel. Start on your knees and reach back with a straight spine so your hands are on the floor just beyond your feet with your fingers facing forwards. From here lift your hips and let your head hang back.

**Take it up a notch** -- If you can easily reach the soles of your feet then have a go at bringing your hands to rest on the floor between your shins.

# Fish

**Fish pose will help to improve your posture by providing a gentle backbend. By drawing your shoulder blades together you create openness in your chest to help you breathe deeper and calm your mind.**

**1.** Begin lying on your back with your hands resting under your buttocks, palms facing down. As you inhale press into your forearms, draw your shoulder blades together and lift your head and torso off the floor. Release your head backwards until the crown of your head lightly rests on the floor.

**2.** Focus on lifting your chest to the sky by drawing your shoulders away from your ears. Gently squeeze your bottom and arch your back throughout the pose to help open the front of your hips.

**3.** To exit the pose, slowly release your head and torso to the ground.

**TARGET AREAS**

**Strengthens:** Upper back and neck
**Stretches:** Hip flexors, belly and chest

**TIPS**

If you feel any discomfort in your head or neck then place a blanket on the floor for your head to rest on.

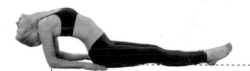

**Variations** -- If your head doesn't reach the floor when you drop it back then allow it to hang back freely so you get a stretch down your throat.

**Take it up a notch** -- To work your core in this pose, lift your legs off the ground and bring your arms in front of you with your palms together so the only areas in contact with the ground are your bottom and your head.

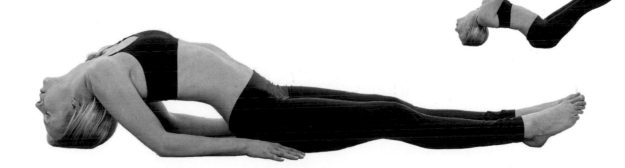

# Flows

**Traditionally in yoga, flows are known as 'vinyasas'. These are breath-synchronised movements that use the mechanical actions of inhalation and exhalation to influence muscular activity, heart rate and the nervous system.**

Moving with the breath in flows assists with flexibility gains by helping you to gauge how much effort and energy you need to bring to each movement. They also help to tune the nervous system for physical activity by increasing blood flow to the muscles and helping you to focus.

Sun Salutations (see p. 116) are the most advanced flows in Yoga Gym and form the basis of many styles of yoga practice. They consist of a series of smooth, flowing movements that take the body through various ranges of motion. Performing them at the beginning of your workout will fire up your nervous system, increase your mobility, and physically and mentally prepare you for the rest of your session.

**BENEFITS OF FLOWS**

Flows take joints through an increasingly greater range of motion to increase flexibility, muscle metabolism and the body's metabolic rate, while triggering the release of toxins. Body temperature is also raised, and by improving the circulation of the synovial fluid in the joints, flows help keep cartilage healthy. Breath and movement are linked while performing the flows, preparing the body for exercise and also drawing awareness to the relationship between the body and the breath.

## HOW TO PERFORM FLOWS

- Focus on matching your movement to your breath and not your breath to your movement.
- Aim to inhale deeply and keep the exhalation long.
- Be patient. Consciously matching your movement to your breath can be tricky to begin with, but as you learn the flows you will naturally adapt to the optimal breathing patterns in the instructions.

# Cat & Cow

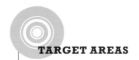

**TARGET AREAS**

Spine, shoulders and wrists

**This is a gentle flow to warm up the spine and prepare you for your workout. Match your movement with your breath as you arch and round your spine to release stress and improve your focus.**

**1.** Begin on all fours with your hands under your shoulders and your knees under your hips.

**2.** Inhale: Dish your back and lift your chest and bottom towards the ceiling. Let your belly drop towards the floor.

**3.** Exhale: Round your back and drop your head. Broaden your shoulder blades around the back of your ribcage. Repeat until your spine feels supple.

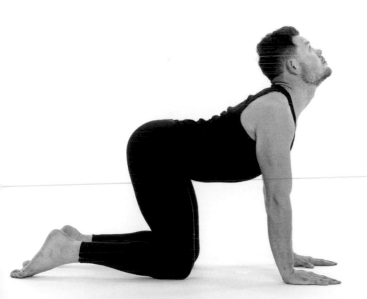

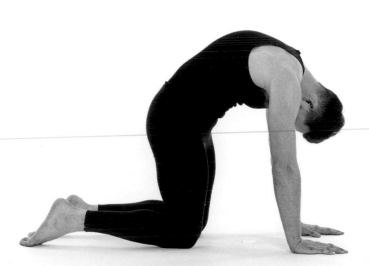

# Eagle Flow

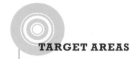
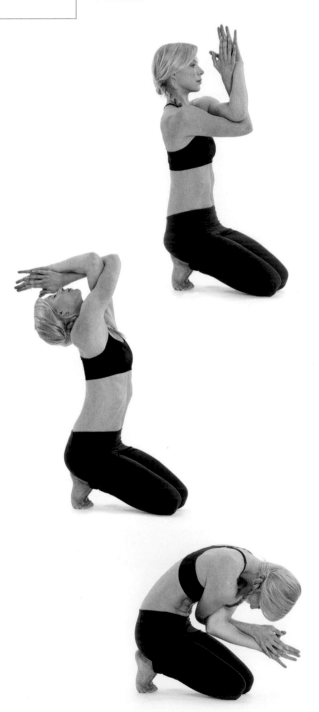

**This is a great way to release tension from your shoulders. You can do it at your desk throughout the day to prevent your from storing stress in your upper body.**

**1.** Begin in a comfortable seated position and bring your arms into Eagle Arms (see p. 77) by crossing your left arm over your right, bending your elbows so your forearms are vertical and then bringing your palms together.

**2.** Inhale: Lift your elbows as high as you can and look up towards the ceiling so you are performing a slight backbend.

**3.** Exhale: Fold forwards by rounding your spine and hug your elbows into your belly to stretch out the back of your shoulders. Repeat until your shoulders feel stress-free and then repeat with the opposite arm on top.

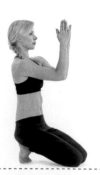

**Variations** -- If you can't get your arms into full Eagle Arms, bring your palms and forearms together in front of you.

# Windshield Wipers

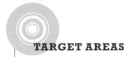
**These rotate the hips both internally and externally to improve mobility. They are great to do in between yin poses as a form of counter pose.**

**1.** Begin seated with your hands resting behind you and your legs bent in front of you with your feet at least hip-width apart.

**2.** Exhale: Let your knees fall to the right, aiming to get both knees touching the floor.

**3.** Inhale: Bring both knees back to centre.

**4.** Repeat to the left, then back and forth from right to left, widening your feet as your hips become more supple.

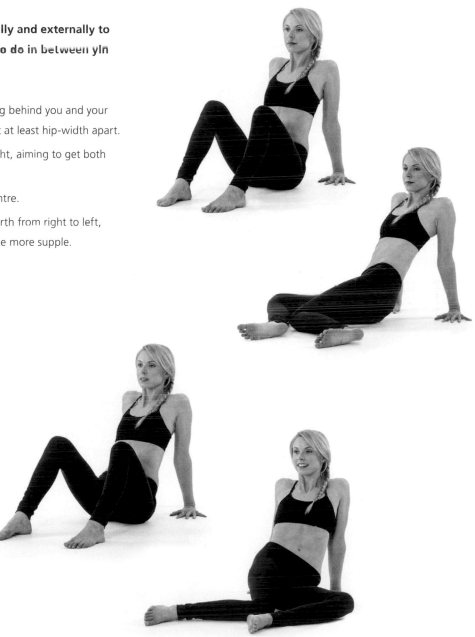

# Forward Bend Flow

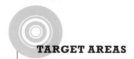

**TARGET AREAS**

Hamstrings, calves and spine

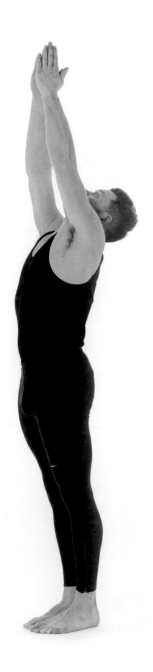

**If you have tight hamstrings this is a gentle way to loosen the backs of your legs. Aim to move with your breath to prepare for the Sun Salutations (see p. 116) and yogacises.**

**1.** Begin standing in Mountain pose (see p. 59) with your feet together or slightly apart and your spine long.

**2.** Inhale: Raise your arms above your head into Prayer Hands (see p. 50).

**3.** Exhale: Fold forwards by hinging from your hips and bringing your fingertips to the floor.

**4.** Inhale: Return to standing and bring your arms above your head. Repeat a few times to release tension from the backs of your legs.

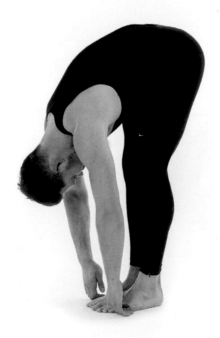

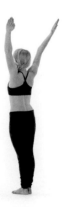

# Y Flow

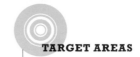
The exercises -- Flows

**This flow moves your shoulders through their full range of motion to reduce any tension and increase flexibility.**

**1.** Begin in Mountain pose (see p. 59) with your spine long and core strong.

**2.** Inhale: Raise your arms above your head to a Y position.

**3.** Exhale: Bring your arms parallel to the floor in front of you with your palms facing each other.

**4.** Inhale: Interlock your fingers and lift your arms above your head so your palms are facing the sky.

**5.** Exhale: Bring your hands behind your head as if you are doing a sit-up.

**6.** Inhale: Reach behind your head to place the palm of each hand on its opposite shoulder.

**7.** Exhale: Release your hands from behind your head and interlock your fingers behind your back.

**8.** Inhale: Push your fingertips to the floor and draw your shoulder blades together.

**9.** Exhale: Bring your hands into Reverse Prayer (see p. 192).

**10.** Inhale: Do a slight backbend making sure you keep your elbows pulled back.

**11.** Exhale: Release your hands from behind your back and bring them above your head with your palms together.

**12.** Inhale: Lean back slightly.

**13.** Exhale: Return to Mountain pose.

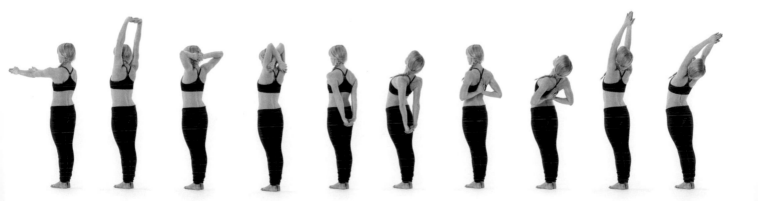

# Sun Salutation A

**TARGET AREAS**

Full body

**TIPS**

Try out the individual poses involved with the Sun Salutation before you attempt the full flow.

Do a round of five Sun Salutations in the morning to get your body and mind energised for the day.

This is a traditional yoga flow that is often used at the start of classes to warm up the body. It encapsulates the essence of yoga in terms of building both strength and flexibility at the same time as being a moving meditation to help you focus for your workout or yoga practice.

**1.** Begin in Mountain pose (see p. 59) with your palms together.

**2.** Inhale: Raise your hands above your head to Upward Salute (see p. 60).

**3.** Exhale: Fold forwards, hinging from your hips, with a long spine to bring your fingertips to the floor.

**4.** Inhale: Lift and lengthen your spine to look straight ahead, leaving your fingertips on the floor.

**5.** Exhale: Step or jump back to Plank (see p. 84) and lower down to Crocodile (see p. 88).

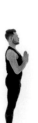 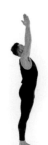   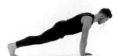 

**6.** Inhale: Lift your chest to Up Dog (see p. 102).

**7.** Exhale: Lift your hips and roll over your toes to Down Dog (see p. 80).

**8.** Breathe here for 5 breaths.

**9.** Exhale: Come up on your toes, soften your knees and look between your hands to Crouching Tiger (see p. 83).

**10.** Inhale: Step or jump your feet in between your hands.

**11.** Exhale: Fold forwards and look to your toes.

**12.** Inhale: Return to standing with your arms above your head.

**13.** Exhale: Release your hands back to Mountain pose.

**Variations** -- You can lower down all the way down to the floor as you build the strength to hover in Crocodile. Feel free to perform Baby Cobra (yang) (see p. 102) instead of Up Dog if you have a stiff spine.

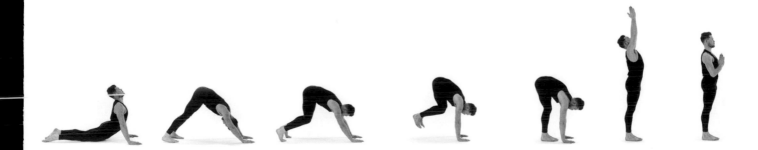

# Sun Salutation B

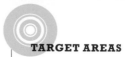
**This is a more advanced version of Sun Salutation A. It works the legs by adding Chair pose (see p. 62) and Warrior 1 (see p. 72) so you get a full-body workout that is focused on building strength in your core, shoulders and thighs.**

**1.** Begin in Mountain pose with your palms together (see p. 59).

**2.** Inhale: Bend your knees, drop your hips and raise your hands above your head with your palms together in Chair.

**3.** Exhale: Straighten your legs as you dive forwards to bring your fingertips to the floor.

**4.** Inhale: Lift and lengthen your spine to look to the front, leaving your fingertips on the floor.

**TIPS**

Perform the Stabilising Sequence (see p. 48) each time you are in Mountain pose. The stronger your core is the easier the transition from Plank to Crocodile will be.

**Perform a few rounds of Sun Salutation A before doing Sun Salutation B, to prepare your body for the movements.**

**Variations** -- If you struggle to step your foot between your hands in preparation for Warrior 1 then you can always take hold of your ankle and drag it forwards.

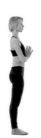
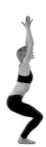

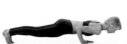

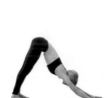
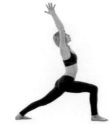
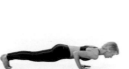
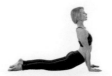
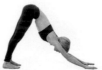

**5.** Exhale: Step or jump back to Plank (see p. 84) and lower down to Crocodile (see p. 88).

**6.** Inhale: Lift your chest to Up Dog (see p. 102).

**7.** Exhale: Lift your hips and roll over your toes to Down Dog (see p. 80).

**8.** Inhale: Step your right foot between your hands and lift your arms above your head to Warrior 1.

**9.** Exhale: Return your palms to the mat either side of your front foot, step back to Plank and lower down to Crocodile.

**10.** Inhale: Lift your chest to Up Dog.

**11.** Exhale: Lift your hips and roll over your toes to Down Dog.

**12.** Inhale: Step your left foot between your hands and lift your arms above your head to Warrior 1.

**13.** Exhale: Return your palms to the mat either side of your front foot, step back to Plank and lower down to Crocodile.

**14.** Inhale: Lift your chest to Up Dog.

**15.** Exhale: Lift your hips and roll over your toes to Down Dog.

**16.** Breathe here for 5 breaths.

**17.** Exhale: Come up on your toes, soften your knees and look between your hands to Crouching Tiger (see p. 83).

**18.** Inhale: Step or jump your feet in between your hands.

**19.** Exhale: Fold forwards and look to your toes.

**20.** Inhale: Bend your knees, drop your hips and lift your arms above your head to Chair pose.

**21.** Exhale: Straighten your legs and release your hands back to Mountain pose.

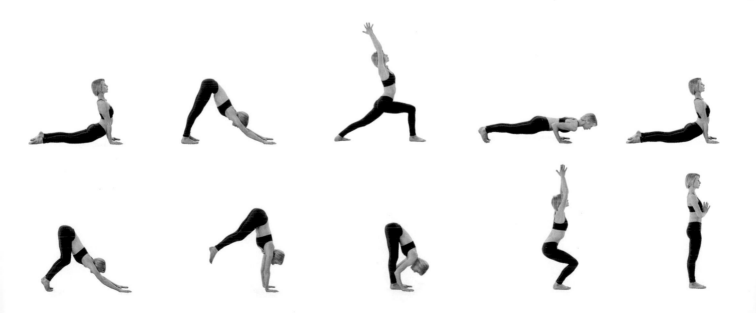

# Rocking Table Top

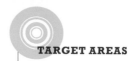

Hips

**This is a great warm-up for the hips and can also be used in between yin poses such as Sleeping Pigeon (see p. 170).**

**1.** Begin on your hands and knees with a neutral spine and take a deep inhale.

**2.** Exhale: Let your hips fall to the right.

**3.** Inhale: Bring your hips back to centre. Repeat to the left. Move right and left until you feel your hips loosening.

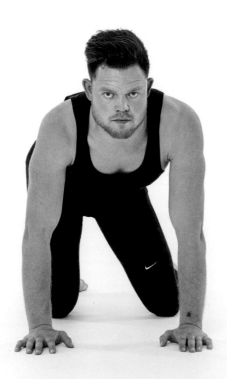
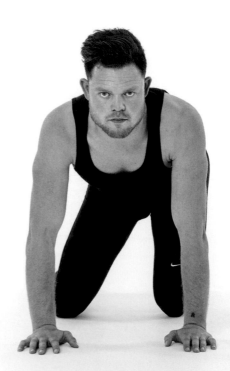

# Yogacises

**Yogacises combine traditional yoga poses with bodyweight exercises to provide an effective way to develop all-round fitness and build an impressive physique.**

The popularity of yoga has brought bodyweight exercise back into fashion. The problem is that yoga alone often fails to build whole-body fitness. Combining traditional yoga poses with yogacises in the Yoga Gym plan provides a systematic way to develop strength, flexibility, power, coordination, cardiovascular endurance, speed and balance.

Yogacises work the whole body rather than isolating certain muscles, as is often the case when using weights. This whole-body approach burns more calories, creates balanced strength and is more demanding on the core. Yogacises also move your body in the way it is designed to move, to keep it functioning properly. By twisting, jumping, pressing, pushing, pulling and moving your body in all sorts of directions, you are mimicking the actions you make in everyday life.

## BENEFITS OF YOGACISES

Yogacises have a profound impact on the body and build fitness on all levels. They consist of compound movements that build strength and power and increase fitness. They increase the heart rate to burn calories, boost the metabolism to promote fat loss, engage the core muscles to enhance posture and athletic performance and improve flexibility by moving the joints through their full range of motion. There is a huge variety to keep exercise interesting and they can be modified to be more or less challenging. They can be done anywhere and are safe for any fitness level.

## HOW TO PERFORM YOGACISES

- Perform the Stabilising Sequence (see p. 48) before each yogacise.
- Move with your breath.
- Make each yogacise slow and steady.
- Follow the instructions carefully to bring your awareness to the areas of the body each yogacise targets.
- Look at Part 3 for an idea of how many repetitions and sets of each yogacise you should do.

# Classic Push-up

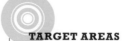

**TARGET AREAS**

**Strengthens:** Chest, arms, shoulders and core

TIPS

If your hips start to sag then repeat the Stabilising Sequence to bring your spine into alignment.

**Lower yourself down slowly with control and then push up as fast and powerfully as possible.**

**Push-ups build strength in the upper body as well as the core. Use the Stabilising Sequence (see p. 48) before you do each push-up to ensure you are moving with proper form.**

**1.** Begin in Plank (see p. 84) with your hands slightly wider than shoulder width. Use the Stabilising Sequence (Bum. Belly. Back: see p. 48) to activate your core and bring your body into alignment.

**2.** Lower yourself down until your chest is hovering just above the floor and your upper arms are parallel to the ground.

**3.** Push back to Plank, keeping your belly braced and your bottom squeezed so your body is in a straight line throughout the entire movement.

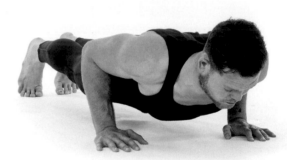

**Variations** -- Building up the strength to do a full push-up takes time. A common variation you see in gyms is dropping your knees to the floor. This changes the angle of your hips so doesn't transfer very well to a proper push-up. A better option is to raise your hands on a surface. You can use a stall, a table, a kitchen worktop, or even push off a wall. As you build strength, slowly lower the surface until you can perform a push-up on the floor.

**Take it up a notch** -- Raise your feet on a stable surface to increase the intensity the yogacise.

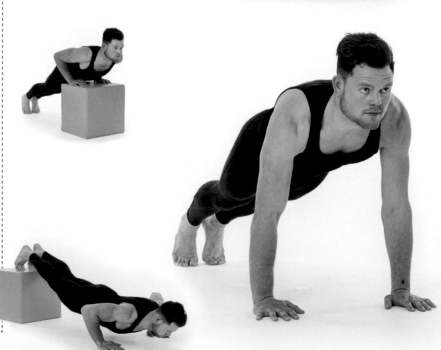

# Narrow Push-up

This is a variation of the Classic Push-up (see p. 122), which targets the backs of your arms. If you want to strengthen your triceps or banish your bingo wings then have a go at these.

**1.** Begin in Plank (see p. 84) pose with your hands slightly less than shoulder-width apart.

**2.** Lower yourself down to Crocodile (see p. 88) until your chest is hovering just above the ground and your upper arms are parallel to the floor.

**3.** Push yourself back to the starting position by straightening your arms.

**TARGET AREAS**

**Strengthens:** Chest, **triceps**, shoulders and core

**TIPS**

Use the Stabilising Sequence (see p. 48) before you begin each repetition to activate your core.

**Variations** -- To make the movement easier, raise your hands on a stable surface.

**Take it up a notch** -- Raise your feet or perform the movement one-legged by lifting one foot off the ground at a time.

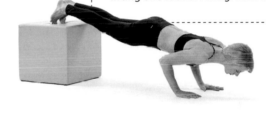

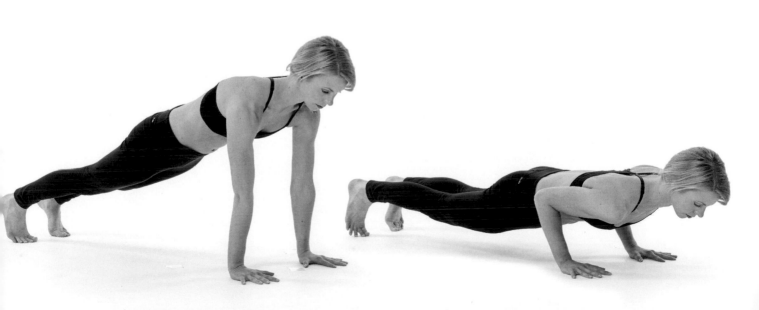

# Yoga Push-up

**Strengthens:** Chest, triceps, shoulders and core

**TIPS**

Move with your breath to ensure each movement is slow and steady.

Aim to get your heels to the ground in Down Dog so that you stretch the backs of your legs.

**A Yoga Push-up is a four-part movement that combines the key postures of Down Dog (see p. 80), Plank (see p. 84) and Crocodile (see p. 88). It's a good idea to feel confident in these poses first so you can move through Yoga Push-ups with correct form.**

**1.** Begin in Down Dog with your hands shoulder-width apart and your feet hip-width apart.

**2.** As you inhale, bring your weight forwards to Plank and as you exhale lower down to Crocodile.

**3.** Inhale and push back up to Plank and exhale back to Down Dog by pushing your bottom to the sky.

**Variations** -- Make the movement easier by raising your hands on a stable surface.

**Take it up a notch** -- Challenge yourself by elevating your feet on a surface. The higher the surface, the more challenging the push-up will be.

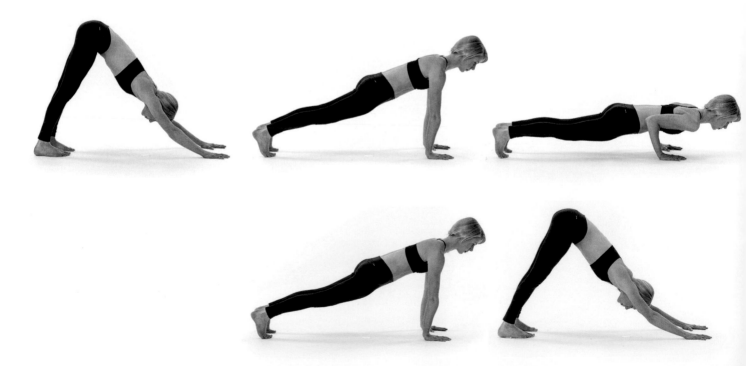

# Crocodile Push-up

**TARGET AREAS**

**Strengthens:** Chest, triceps, shoulders and core

**TIPS**

Move your body as one unit rather than seeing it as separate limbs.

If you find your hips are sagging then think about pushing your lower back to the sky.

Crocodile Push-ups use isometric as well as dynamic muscle contraction. By pausing at the top of the movement in Crocodile pose (see p. 88) you will be strengthening both the agonist and antagonist muscles to enable you to hold the pose statically.

**1.** Begin lying on your belly with your elbows bent and palms on the floor in line with your chest. Hook your toes under, lift your chest and lift your kneecaps.

**2.** Lift your hips off the floor to Crocodile, then use the Stabilising Sequence (see p. 48) to stabilise your pelvis and hold for 3 breaths.

**3.** Lower yourself back down to the ground, keeping your spine in a straight line.

**Variations** -- Raise your hips on a block or cushion to help you build up to the full movement.

**Take it up a notch** -- Rather than increasing the intensity of the yogacise, increase the duration. Build up the amount of time you hold Crocodile pose for 5 to 10 breaths.

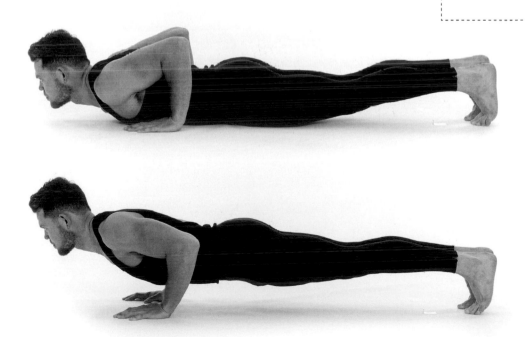

# Bouncing Push-up

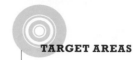

**Strengthens:** Shoulders, arms, core and wrists

**This is the same as the Classic Push-up (see p. 122), but you push your hands off the floor at the top of the movement to build explosive power. We often don't know how powerful our body is until we perform movements like this, so focus on where you can transfer that power to in other areas of training and life.**

**1.** Begin in Plank (see p. 84) with your arms straight and core tight.

**2.** Lower your chest down to the ground, as you would in a Classic Push-up.

**3.** Push yourself up as fast as you can so your hands leave the ground, keeping your spine straight. Land as gently as you can back in Plank, softening your elbows and finding your balance with your fingertips.

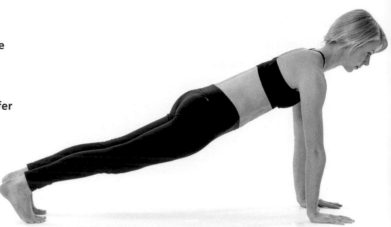

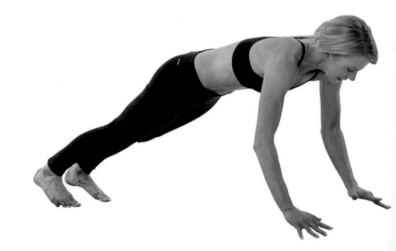

**Variations** -- It doesn't matter if your hands don't leave the ground to begin with. Pushing up as fast as you can will build the power you need to get off the floor.

**Take it up a notch** -- Pause at the bottom of the movement before you explode back up again.

**TIPS**

Keep your elbows tucked into your body rather than letting them wing out.

**Land on your fingertips and then your palms to soften your landing.**

# Down Dog Push-up

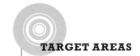

**TARGET AREAS**

**Strengthens:** Arms and shoulders

**TIPS**

Pull up on your kneecaps and engage the fronts of your thighs to keep your legs straight.

**If you want to master arm balances such as Handstand and Forearm Stand (see p. 194) then Down Dog Push-ups will build the strength you need in your shoulders.**

**1.** Begin in Down Dog (see p. 80) with your hands shoulder-width apart and your heels as close to the ground as possible.

**2.** Bend your elbows until your head touches the floor. Keep you back straight throughout the entire movement. Only your arms should move.

**3.** Push back to Down Dog by straightening your arms.

**Variations** -- Raise your hands on an elevated surface to make the yogacise easier. Slowly lower the height of the surface as you get stronger.

**Take it up a notch** -- Place your feet on a raised surface to make the yogacise more challenging.

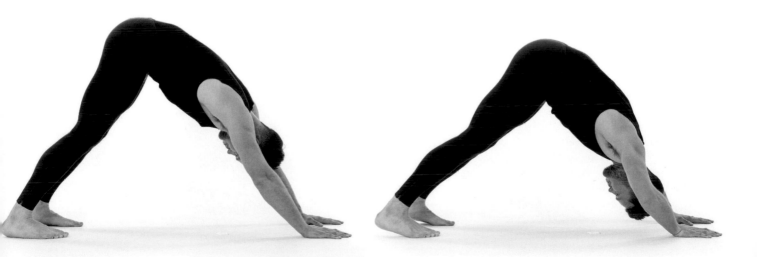

# Windmill Push-up

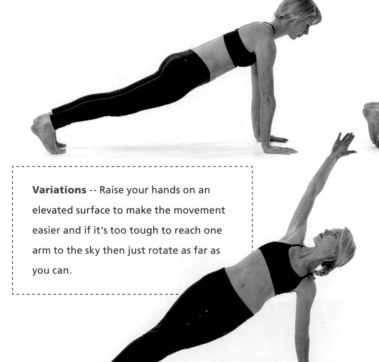

**TARGET AREAS**

**Strengthens:** Arms, shoulders and core

**TIPS**

Focus on twisting from your core, allowing your chest, shoulders and head to follow.

Draw your shoulder blades together as you reach your hands to the sky to help deepen the twist.

Windmill Push-ups take the Classic Push-up to a new level by adding in a twist to strengthen the core. As always, take the yogacise at your own pace and pick from the variations below to suit your fitness level.

**1.** Begin in Plank (see p. 84).

**2.** Lower yourself down to Crocodile (see p. 88).

**3.** Push back up to Plank and rotate from your core to lift your right hand to the sky. Place your right hand back on the ground in Plank. Alternate which way you rotate and which hand you lift with every repetition.

**Take it up a notch** -- Make the yogacise more challenging by placing a medicine ball or football under the hand of the arm that you're not lifting. Just switch the ball when you're in Plank, halfway through the repetition.

**Variations** -- Raise your hands on an elevated surface to make the movement easier and if it's too tough to reach one arm to the sky then just rotate as far as you can.

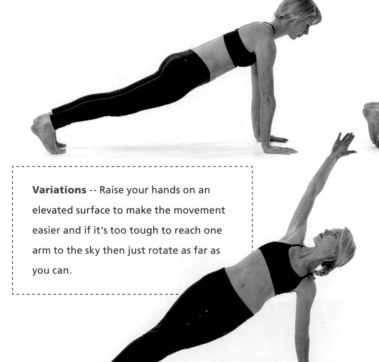

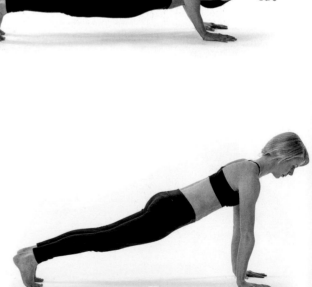

# Rocking Plank

**TARGET AREAS**

**Strengthens:** Shoulders, core and wrists

Rocking Plank is a simple exercise but that doesn't mean it's easy. It requires body awareness, core strength and wrist flexibility.

**1.** Begin in Plank (see p. 84) with your arms straight and core tight.

**2.** Use your toes to push your body forwards to Planche Plank (see p. 86) so your shoulders move between one and two hand lengths in front of your wrists.

**3.** Push back to Plank, bringing your shoulders directly above your wrists.

**TIPS**

Look at the ground straight ahead of you throughout the movement to help keep your spine in line.

**Push your weight into the area where your index finger joins your palms to help ease any wrist pain.**

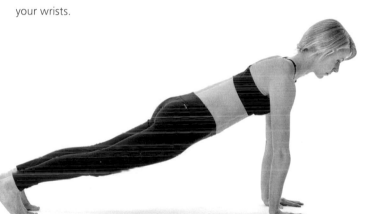

**Variations** -- If your wrists feel under pressure in this yogacise, try rotating your hands so your fingers are facing out to the side or back towards your toes.

**Take it up a notch** -- If you find this easy then add in a Classic Push-up after you've moved your body forwards.

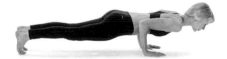

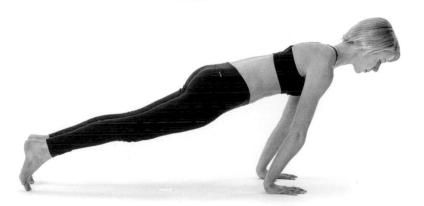

# Down Dog Bomber

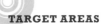

**Strengthens:** Chest, shoulders, arms and core

Down Dog Bombers are great to do to build up strength for the Sun Salutations (see p. 116). They strengthen the entire upper body as well as increasing flexibility in the spine and developing pure core strength.

**1.** Begin in Down Dog (see p. 80) with your hands shoulder-width apart and your feet hip-width apart.

**2.** Bend your elbows into your sides and swoop your chest forwards through Crocodile (see p. 88) before straightening your arms to Up Dog (see p. 102).

**3.** Reverse the movement by bending your elbows and lowering your chest to the floor to Crocodile and then pushing your bottom to the sky to Down Dog.

**TIPS**

Arch your back in Up Dog to restore mobility in the spine and stretch out your belly.

Keep your core strong throughout the movement so you are not moving your upper and lower body as two separate units.

**Variations** -- If you find reversing the movement too tough to begin with then lift your hips and roll over your toes straight from Up Dog to Down Dog.

**Take it up a notch** -- If you find this easy then lift one foot off the ground, alternating legs for each repetition.

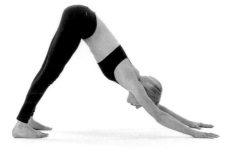
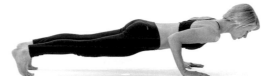
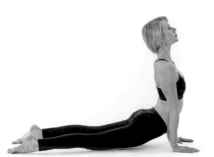
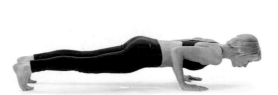
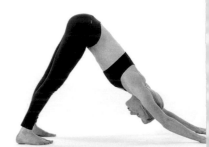

# Bear Crawl

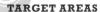

**TARGET AREAS**

**Strengthens:** Shoulders, biceps, triceps and upper back

**TIPS**

Take this yogacise outside and do it in the garden if you can. Kids love to join in with it too.

Make sure you look where you're going so you don't bump into anything!

Crawling is one of the most basic forms of movement. From the age of a few months old we are on our hands and knees getting to know our body and learning how to move it. After years of sitting behind desks, in cars and on sofas, we can lose this connection. The Bear Crawl re-establishes this primal movement, building strength in the upper body and restoring optimal movement patterns.

**1.** Begin in Table Top (see p. 78) and lift your knees off the ground to Bear pose (see p. 79).

**2.** Propel yourself forwards on all fours for 30 seconds without letting your knees touch the ground. If you run out of space then move sideways and backwards too.

**3.** Lower your knees to the ground and rest in Table Top.

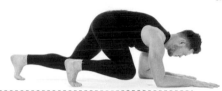

**Take it up a notch** -- To make the movement more challenging, bring your forearms to the floor as you do in Dolphin pose (see p. 82) and crawl around on your feet and forearms.

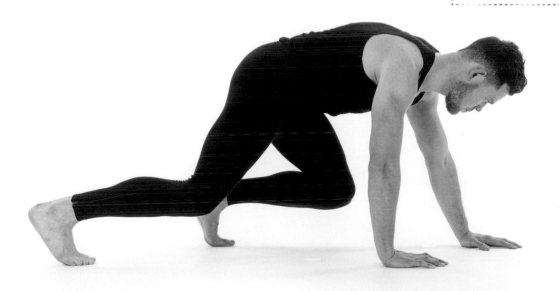

# Crab Walk

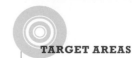
**Strengthens:** Back and triceps

**This is moving version of Reverse Table Top (see p. 103), which targets your whole posterior chain, especially your triceps.**

**TIPS**

Squeeze your bottom muscles to prevent your hips sagging.

**1.** Begin in Reverse Table Top with your shoulders above your wrists.

**2.** Walk forwards, backwards and sideways for 30 seconds, keeping your hips as high as possible.

**3.** Lower your bottom to the ground and massage out the backs of your hands if necessary.

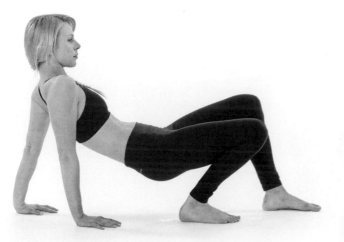
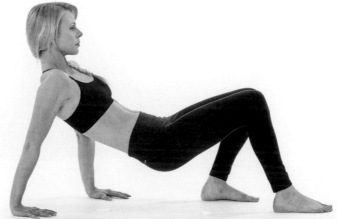

# Squat

Squatting is one of the most fundamental human movements. We use it in everyday activities, such as getting up from a chair, as well as in athletic actions such as jumping. Squatting is a dynamic combination of Chair pose (see p. 62) and Toddler Squat (see p. 166) and works the biggest muscles in your body to build strength, stabilise the core and sculpt your thighs.

**1.** Stand with your feet about hip-width apart. Have your toes pointing straight forwards or turned out slightly. Use the Stabilising Sequence (see p. 48) to stabilise your pelvis and bring your spine into optimal alignment.

**2.** Bend your knees and push your hips back as if you are sitting on a chair, then lower yourself until your bottom is between your heels.

**3.** Stand up by pushing your weight into your feet and straightening your legs, making sure you keep your heels on the floor.

**Variations** -- If you can't sit all the way down between your heels then aim to get your thighs parallel to the floor to begin with.

**Take it up a notch** -- Make the squat more challenging by pausing in the bottom position for 1–10 seconds.

**TARGET AREAS**

**Strengthens:** Thighs, bottom, lower back and hips

**TIPS**

Lean your upper body slightly forwards as you lower yourself down to help you balance.

Push your weight back into your heels and keep your knees out to ensure proper form.

The exercises -- Yogacises

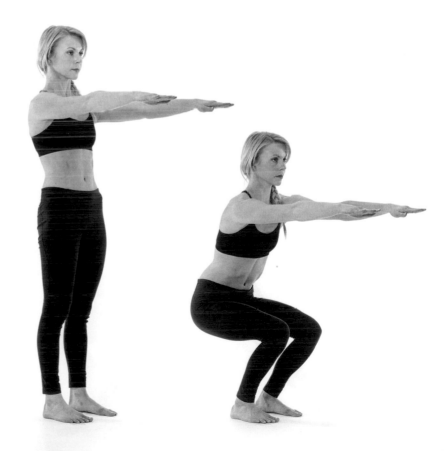

135

# Squat Jump

**Strengthens:** Thighs, bottom, lower back, calves and hips

Adding a jump to the squat builds strength and power. Explosive yogacises such as these get your body moving quickly, develop fast-twist muscle fibres and increase your metabolism. Explode as quickly as you can from the bottom position to see the best results.

**1.** Begin in Mountain pose (see p. 59) with your feet about hip-width apart.

**2.** Bend your knees and sink your hips until your bottom touches your heels.

**3.** Explode forcefully from the bottom position, jumping as high as possible and landing softly with your feet hip-width apart.

Lower yourself down to the bottom position with control so you can find your balance before you explode upwards.

**Cushion your landing by softening your knees as your feet touch the floor.**

Squeeze your buttocks and extend your hips as you jump upwards to develop strength in the rear of your body.

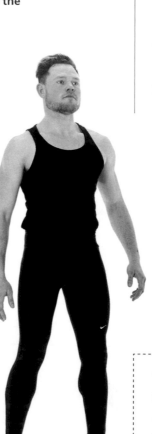

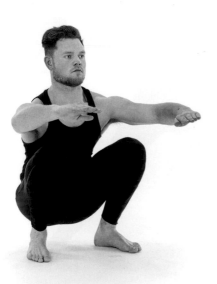

**Variations** -- If you can't get your bottom all the way to your heels then do Half or Quarter Squat Jumps with your knees bent between 45 and 90 degrees.

**Take it up a notch** -- Make the Squat Jump more challenging by pausing in the bottom position for 1–10 seconds so you are using pure explosive power rather than the stretch reflex.

# Star Jump

**This is one of the best exercises for building shapely buttocks. You probably remember doing Star Jumps on the school field as a child so your body will recognise the movement and it will begin to flow naturally after a few repetitions.**

**1.** Begin with your feet spread wide and your knees bent out to the side in Sun God pose (see p. 63). Bring your hands to the floor in between your feet and look straight ahead.

**2.** Explode upwards, stretching your arms and legs as wide as possible into a star shape.

**3.** Descend back to the ground and land softly in the starting position.

## TARGET AREAS

**Strengthens:** Thighs, bottom, calves and hips

**TIPS**

Cushion your descent by landing on your toes before spreading your weight on to your heels.

**Squeeze your bottom as you jump to help widen your legs and stretch your inner thighs.**

**Variations** -- If you struggle with Sun God pose and Sumo Squats (see p. 136), an alternative is to begin and end each Star Jump in Mountain pose (see p. 59).

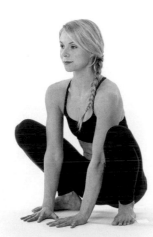
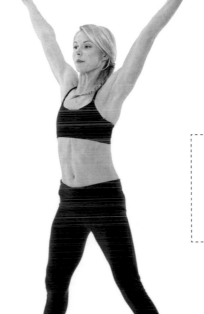

# Lunge

**Strengthens:** Thighs and bottom

**TIPS**

Distribute your weight evenly across both feet to help you balance.

**Not all actions we do in life involve our feet being side by side, and Lunges work your muscles in lines that are used for walking and running rather than sitting and standing. By splitting your legs, you can focus on working one side of your body at a time to reduce any muscular imbalances.**

**Take it up a notch** -- Make the Lunge more challenging by pausing in the bottom position for 1–10 seconds.

**1.** Stand in Mountain pose (see p. 59) and take a big step forwards with your right foot. Come up on to the toes of your left foot and perform the Stabilising Sequence (see p. 116) to ensure your buttocks are firm, belly is braced and spine is supported.

**2.** Bend your knees and sink your hips so that you left knee almost touches the ground.

**3.** Push through the heel of your right foot, straighten your leg, and step your right foot back to Mountain pose. Repeat the exercise as many times as required, finishing your set on the right leg. Repeat with your left foot forwards.

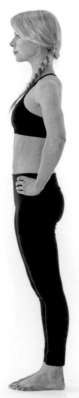
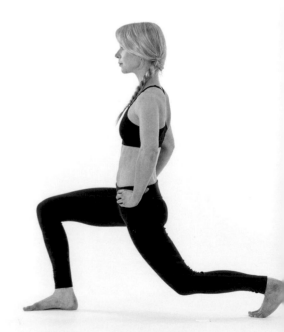

# Reverse Lunge

## TARGET AREAS

**Strengthens:** Thighs and bottom

This is the same as a normal Lunge, only you're stepping backwards instead of forwards. Many people find the Reverse Lunge easier because your centre of gravity is kept between your two feet and it puts less stress on the knee joint. It is still a challenging yogacise though, as it gives the body the opportunity to work in a direction it doesn't usually travel in – backwards.

**TIPS**

Aim to create a 90-degree angle at both knees so that your front shin and back thigh are perpendicular to the ground.

Time your breathing with your movements so you are inhaling and exhaling on the descent and ascent.

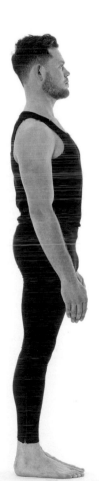

**1.** Stand in Mountain pose (see p. 59) and take a big step backwards with your right foot.

**2.** Bend your knees and sink your hips so that you right knee almost touches the ground.

**3.** Push yourself up and step your feet together. Repeat the exercise as many times as necessary, finishing your set on your right leg. Repeat the same number of repetitions stepping your left foot back.

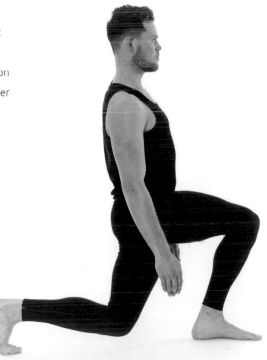

# Power Lunge

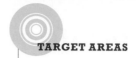

**Strengthens:** Thighs and bottom

**The Power Lunge builds explosive strength so you will develop muscular force for other types of exercises. It combines the Reverse Lunge (see p. 141) with a powerful hop to build balance and stability as well as strengthening and toning the thighs.**

**1.** Begin in the Reverse Lunge position with your right foot back and your right knee almost touching the floor.

**2.** With as much power as possible, shoot your right knee forwards and up towards your chest as you hop as high as you can on your left foot.

**3.** Land softly on your left foot and sweep you right leg behind you to return to your starting position. Repeat the exercise as many times as necessary, then switch legs.

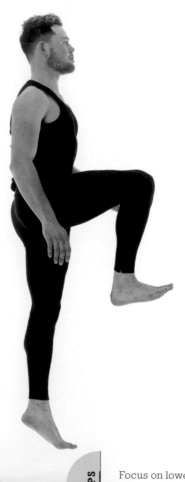

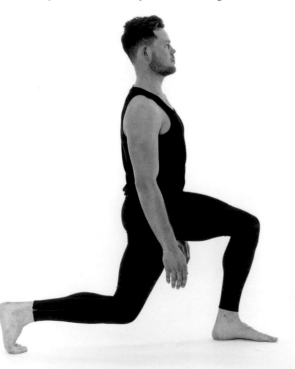

**TIPS**

Focus on lowering back to Reverse Lunge slowly and with control and then jumping up as fast as you can.

142

# Split Squat

**TARGET AREAS**

**Strengthens:** Thighs and bottom

**If you want an alternative to Lunges (see p. 140) then Split Squats are a good option. You still work your thighs and your buttocks without having to focus so much on your balance. Make sure you keep your core tight and bottom squeezed throughout the yogacise to achieve full extension of the hips.**

**TIPS**

Aim to keep your hips in line throughout the movement so your spine stays in alignment.

Notice how squeezing your bottom and bracing your belly makes the movement more stable.

**1.** Stand in Mountain pose (see p. 59) and take a big step forwards with your right foot. Come up on to the toes of your left foot and perform the Stabilising Sequence (see p. 116) to ensure your buttocks are firm, belly is braced and spine is supported.

**Variations** -- You can begin with your front foot on a step to make the Split Squat easier.

**2.** Bend your knees and sink your hips so that you right knee almost touches the ground and both knees are at a right angle.

**3.** Push through the heel of your right foot and straighten both legs without locking your knees to return to your split leg starting position. Finish all repetitions with your right leg forwards before repeating on the left leg.

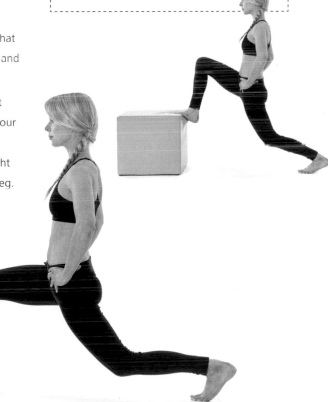

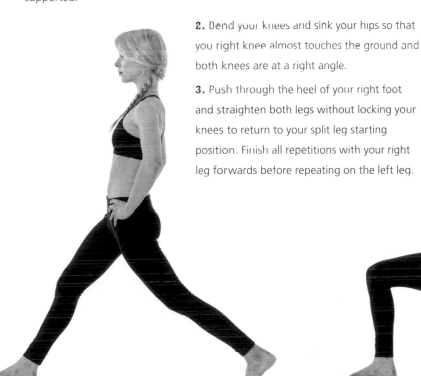

# Half Moon Bend

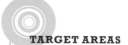

**TARGET AREAS**

**Strengthens:** Core, waist and lower back

**TIPS**

Keep your elbows glued to your ears and your elbows straight to develop muscular endurance in your arms.

**Keep your bottom squeezed and core strong throughout the movement to emphasise lateral flexion.**

**Just like Half Moon pose (see p. 61), Half Moon Bends build strength in the core and increase flexibility in the spine. It is a great yogacise to correct your posture by building stability in your lower back and abdominals and stretching out the entire side of your body.**

**1.** Begin in Mountain pose (see p. 59) and reach your arms above your head as you inhale to Upward Salute (see p. 60).

**2.** Exhale and fold to the right by hinging from your hip and engaging the underside of your body.

**3.** As you inhale, return to centre using the strength of your core. That is one repetition. Repeat to the left and then alternate which side you fold to for the remaining repetitions.

**Variations** -- If your shoulders ache when you have your palms together then position your hands about shoulder-width apart above your head.

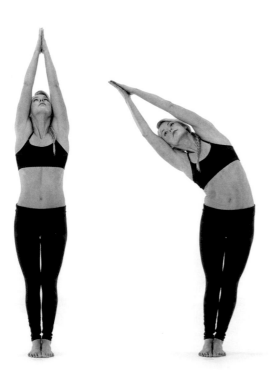
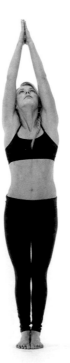
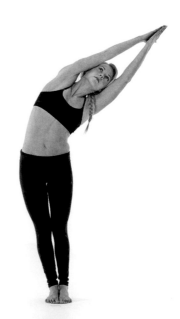

# Iron Cross

**TARGET AREAS**

**Strengthens:** Core and waist

TIPS

Exhale as you lower your legs to relieve any tension in your lower back.

**Focus on lowering your legs down slowly and steadily.**

**Iron Crosses add a dynamic element to yang-style twists. They force your core muscles to work to build stability as you move to create a defined waist. This is also a wonderful way to release any tension from the back and help your spine to unwind.**

**1.** Begin lying on your back and spread your arms out to the side. Raise your legs so your toes are pointing towards the sky.

**2.** Keeping your body in an L shape and your hips at a 90-degree angle, lower your legs down to the right by twisting from your waist as you exhale. Stop when your feet are hovering just above the floor, making sure both shoulder blades remain in contact with the ground.

**3.** As you inhale, bring your legs back to centre. That is one repetition. Lower your legs to the left and return to centre and then continue alternating the side to which you lower your legs for the remaining repetitions.

**Variations** -- Bend your knees to make the yogacise easier.

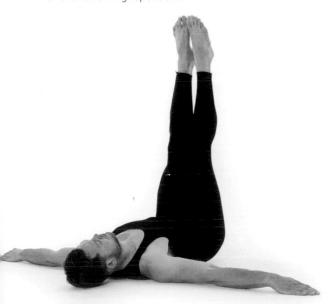
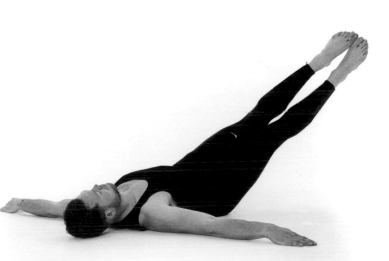

# Rocking Boat

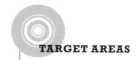

**Strengthens:** Core and hip flexors

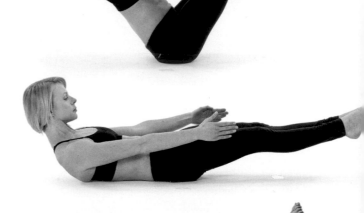

**The Rocking Boat yogacise is a total core-working movement that challenges your abs, back, hip flexors and thighs. It's often called a V-up or Jack-knife Sit-up and adds a dynamic element to Boat pose (see p. 89) to build core strength and sculpt your abs.**

**1.** Begin in Boat pose so only your bottom is touching the floor with your arms stretched out in front of you.

**2.** Slowly lower your chest back and your legs down to Low Boat pose (see p. 90) as you inhale, so your shoulders and feet are just above the ground.

**3.** As you exhale, hinge from your hips to lift your legs and torso back to Boat pose.

**Variations** -- This is a challenging ab exercise so an alternative is to begin in Baby Boat (see p. 89) with your legs bent and straighten your legs as you lower down to Low Boat. Return to Baby Boat by bending your legs as you lift your chest.

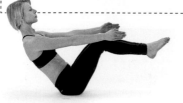

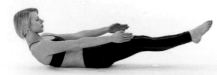

**TIPS**

Look up and over your toes in Boat pose to keep your spine long.

**Let your shoulders relax away from your ears to lengthen your spine and prevent you from wasting energy.**

# Triple Down Dog

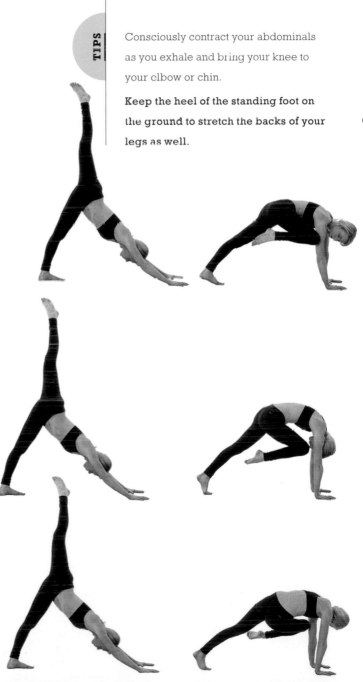

**TARGET AREAS**

**Strengthens:** Core, waist and shoulders

**TIPS**

Consciously contract your abdominals as you exhale and bring your knee to your elbow or chin.

Keep the heel of the standing foot on the ground to stretch the backs of your legs as well.

**Triple Down Dogs work the whole body to improve coordination at the same time as strengthening the core. Optimal breathing patterns have a powerful effect on this yogacise, so focus on moving with each inhalation and each exhalation.**

**1.** Begin in Down Dog (see p. 80) and step your feet together. Lift your right foot to the sky into Three-legged Dog (see p. 81).

**2.** On an exhalation, bring your right knee to your right elbow as you shift your weight forwards to bring your shoulders over your wrists, and as you inhale kick your leg back to Three-legged Dog.

**3.** Exhale as you repeat the movement, but this time bring your knee to your chin. Pause for a moment and return to Three-legged Dog as you inhale. Repeat a third time but this time add a twist as your bring your right knee to your left elbow and then kick back to Three-legged Dog as you inhale. That is one repetition. Complete your required repetitions and repeat with the left leg.

# Hip-up

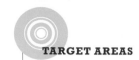

**TARGET AREAS**

**Strengthens:** Core, hamstrings and shoulders

**TIPS**

Focus on creating a straight line from your shoulders to your knees.

Draw your shoulder blades together at the top of the Hip-up to stretch the front of your chest.

**This is a full-body exercise with a focus on strengthening the core. Prepare for it by performing Reverse Table Top (see p. 103) so your body learns the posture in the top position.**

**1.** Begin seated with your legs bent and your feet on the floor in front of you. Reach your arms back on the floor with your fingers pointing forwards. Inhale as you focus on lengthening your spine.

**2.** Push your weight evenly into your hands and feet and lift your hips until your spine is parallel to the floor and your knees are at a right angle. Squeeze your buttocks at the top and hold for 3 seconds.

**3.** Lower back to the starting position slowly.

> **Take it up a notch** -- Lift one leg off the floor and perform One-legged Hip-ups.

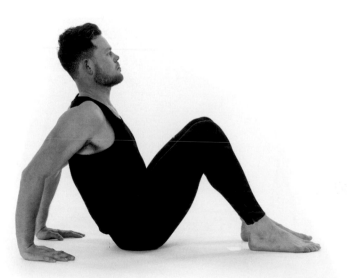

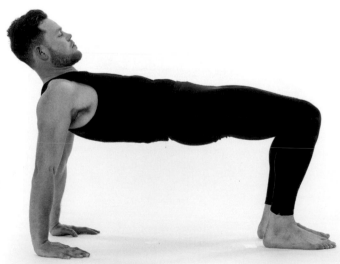

# Locust Lift

**Strengthens:** Bottom and lower back

Locust lifts develop both strength and flexibility in the lower back. Like Locust pose (see p. 105) it is a **hyperextension** movement that targets the **erector spinae** – the columns of muscles that run parallel to the spine. Balance out this extension of the spine with Rocking Boats (see p. 154) or Low Boat pose (see p. 90) to keep the body in balance.

**TIPS**

Pad the floor beneath your hips with a cushion or blanket to provide some padding your pelvis and ribs.

Stabilise your lower back by pushing your pubic bone in the floor before you lift.

1. Begin lying on your belly with your arms beside you.

2. Lift your legs and arms off the ground to Locust pose and hold for 3 seconds.

3. Lower back down to the starting position. That is one repetition.

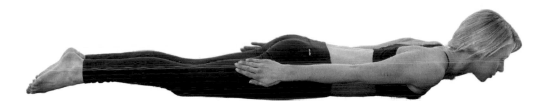

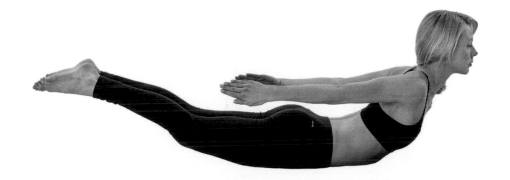

# Yogic Bicycles

**Strengthens:** Core and waist

This is one of the most effective ab exercises, which combines Low Boat pose (see p. 90) with a dynamic twist to strengthen the core and define the waist.

(see p. 90)

**1.** Begin in Low Boat pose and press your lower back towards the floor.

**2.** Bring your right knee into your chest and reach your left elbow to the outside of your right knee as you exhale.

**3.** Straighten out your right knee and bend your left knee to your chest as you twist your torso to bring your right elbow to the outside of your left knee. That is one repetition.

**TIPS**

Focus on making the movements slow and controlled rather than rushing through the set.

**Consciously contract your abs as you bring your elbow to the outside of your knee.**

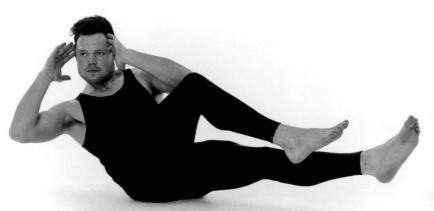
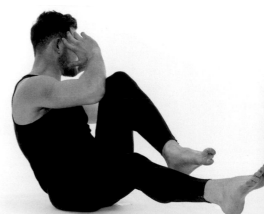

# Crunch

**TARGET AREAS**

**Strengthens:** Bottom and lower back

**TIPS**

This is not a sit-up: it is a crunch. By only lifting until your fingertips touch your knees you are avoiding placing strain on your lower back.

**Crunches are an old favourite when it comes to ab exercises, but it's important you do them properly. Many people hold their breath, go too quickly or use their neck or back muscles to pull them up. Make sure you breathe as you move, keep the crunch slow and steady and use the strength of your core.**

**1.** Lie on your back and bend your knees to bring the soles of your feet to the floor. Push your lower back towards the floor, keeping the natural curve in your spine. Reach your hands out in front of you and rest your palms on your thighs. Draw your belly button towards the floor and use the strength of your core to raise your torso just enough so you can touch your knees with your fingertips.

**2.** Lower yourself back down to the ground until your shoulder blades touch the floor.

**Variations** -- To make this exercise easier, hook your toes under a stable object such as a bed or sofa.

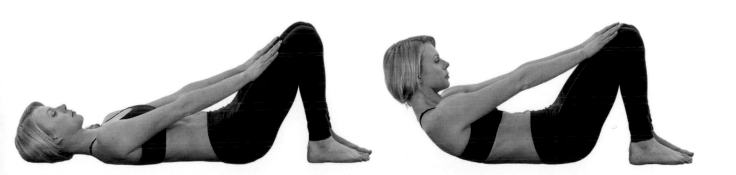

# Flutter Kicks

**Strengthens:** Core and hip flexors

**TIPS**

Keep your legs straight by pulling up on your kneecaps and engaging your quadriceps.

You can do the yogacise quickly or slowly, but make sure each movement is mindful.

**A Flutter Kick is a simple and effective yogacise that builds strength and endurance in the muscles in your lower abs and at the front of your hips. It is a great yogacise to do at the end of a workout as a finisher exercise to really challenge yourself.**

**1.** Lie on your back and place your hands underneath your bottom. Lift your legs off the ground as if you are doing Low Boat pose (see p. 90) but leave your upper body on the floor.

**2.** Lift your right leg about 12.5cm (5in) and then lower it in line with your left leg.

**3.** Lift your left leg about 12.5cm (5in) and then lower it in line with your right leg. That is one repetition.

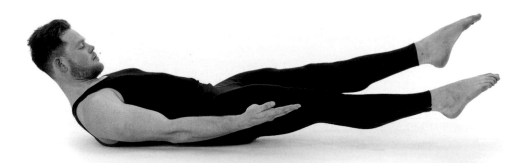

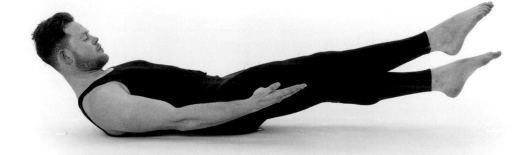

# Floating Straddle

TARGET AREAS

**Strengthens:** Core and hip flexors

This combines the core strengthening aspects of Low Boat pose (see p. 90) with the flexibility-inducing elements of a Seated Wide Leg Forward Bend (see p. 95). By opening and closing your legs in a controlled movement, you strengthen the outside of your hips as well as your abs.

**TIPS**

You can raise your head off the floor to strengthen your neck.

**Notice how squeezing your bottom helps to widen your Straddle.**

Push your lower back towards the floor to keep your spine in alignment.

**1.** Lie on your back with your hands under your bottom. Lift your feet about 15cm (6in) off the ground so your lower body is in the same shape as Low Boat.

**2.** Open your legs as wide as possible to Straddle position (see p. 169).

**3.** Bring your feet together and squeeze your knees together.

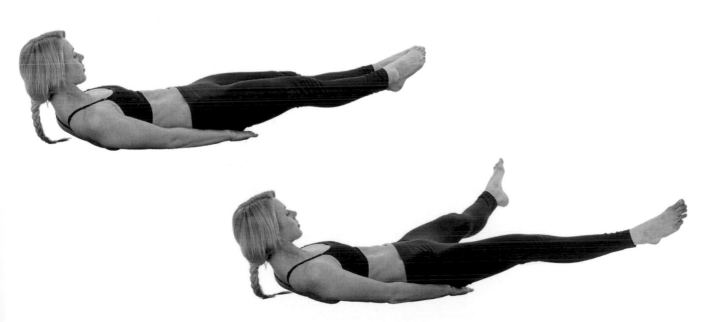

# Yin poses

**Yin poses are passive and relaxing. Most of us live fast-paced and often stressful lifestyles. Combine this with challenging yang poses, yogacises and other types of exercise and an imbalance is created, which is why we need yin poses.**

Yin poses are simple but also very challenging. They target the yin tissues (fascia, ligaments and tendons, rather than the yang tissues – muscles, blood and skin) and joints. This results in optimal mobility and strengthens the connective tissues. Each pose is held from 1 to 20 minutes to give the body time and space to open. Unlike muscles, which are elastic and respond well to the rhythmic movements of flows, yogacises and yang poses, connective tissues require a slow and gentle approach.

Rather than actively stretching and strengthening muscles as you do in yang poses, in yin poses the aim is to relax the muscles so we can target the joints. By stressing (not stretching) the connective tissues around the joints, the tissues will become longer, thicker and stronger over time. It is important not to use yang movements on yin tissues. Only with the long, gentle pressure of yin poses can yin tissues be strengthened and optimal mobility regained.

Yin poses can have a profound impact on our mental state too. By bringing our awareness inwards to our breath and the different sensations in our body during each pose, we will be able to notice changes in our emotional state as the yin nature of the poses brings a wholeness to our practice and unity to body, mind and heart. If you want to find out more about the philosophy on yin yoga then I highly recommend reading the work of Sarah Powers, Bernie Clark and Paul Grilley.

## HOW TO PERFORM YIN POSES

- Move into the pose to an appropriate depth where you feel significant resistance, stretch, compression or twist – this is known as your edge.
- Play your edge and move deeper into the pose as your body opens.
- Remain still in the pose once you have found your edge to keep the muscles inactive, so you are targeting your joints.
- Hold the pose from 1–20 minutes, depending on the pose, by building the hold time up slowly. The hold times in this book are written as a number of breaths so you don't have to clock watch. Aim to do 6–10 breaths per minute.
- Keep your focus on your breath to prevent your mind from wandering.
- Slight discomfort in yin poses is normal, but if you feel pain or tingling in the fingers or toes then come out of the pose slowly.

# Benefits of yin poses

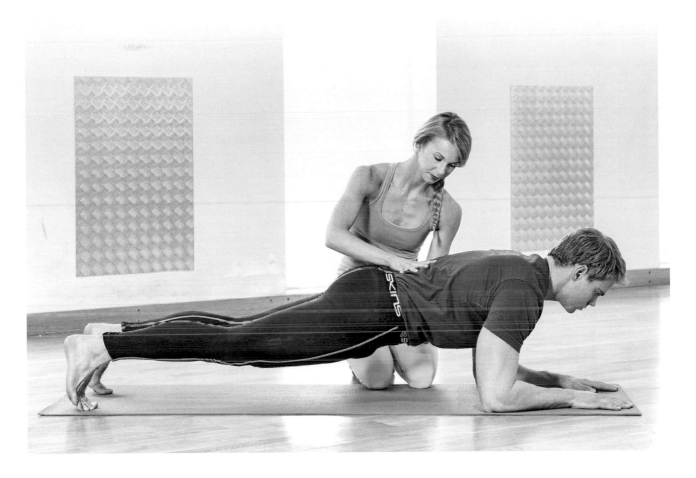

Yin poses help to improve flexibility by realigning muscle fibres in the fascia. They also increase range of motion by stimulating fibroblast growth and hydrate tissues and joints. Connective tissues are strengthened by the increased collagen production, and by working on the joints, yin poses help re-establish healthy spinal curves for optimal posture and movement. In addition to fibroblasts, osteoblasts, the cells that make bones, are also stimulated, which can help prevent bone degeneration that often occurs with age.

Performing yin poses also has many non-physical benefits, as it calms the body and mind, improves mindfulness by bringing awareness to the present moment and releases energy blockages trapped in the body.

# Ragdoll

**Stretches:** Hamstrings, back and calves
**Hold Time:** 10–30 breaths

**Ragdoll loosens the hamstrings and releases any tension from the lower back. Use as little muscular effort as possible so that your body can work with gravity to completely relax into the pose.**

**1.** Start standing with your feet about hip-width apart. Soften your knees and slowly roll forwards one vertebrae at a time. Allow your spine to round and your head to hang. Take hold of the opposite elbow and dangle passively.

**2.** Allow gravity to help you fold forwards to release tension from your lower back and hamstrings. Let your head hang loosely and relax your elbows closer to the floor with each exhalation.

**3.** To come out of the pose, release your hands to the floor and slowly roll back up to standing.

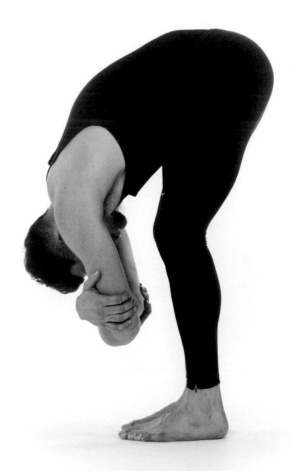

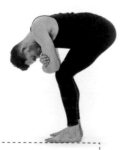

**Variations** -- If you feel tightness in your back or hamstrings then bend your knees more and rest your elbows on your thighs.

**Take it up a notch** -- If you are already flexible then take hold of your elbows behind your thighs.

**TIPS**

Allow yourself to dangle passively in this pose and sway gently from side to side if that feels good.

# Wide Squat

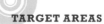

**TARGET AREAS**

**Stretches:** Hips, inner thighs, lower back and ankles

**Hold Time:** 5–30 breaths

**TIPS**

Flow between Wide Squat and Ragdoll (see p. 164) to release tension from the lower back.

This is a lovely way to stretch the inner thighs, release tension from the hips, and increase mobility in the pelvis. Many people find it challenging to relax into the pose to begin with, so start holding the pose for 5 breaths and build it up to 30 breaths as your mind–muscle connection improves and your flexibility increases.

**1.** Begin standing with your feet slightly wider than hip-width apart. Turn your toes outwards about 45 degrees. Squat down to bring your bottom between your heels and bring your hands in front of you with your hands in Prayer Hands (see p. 50) and your elbows resting on your inner thighs.

**2.** Focus on relaxing your heels and keeping your knees out to stretch the inner thighs.

**3.** To exit the pose, slowly straighten your legs to return to standing.

**Variations** -- If your heels are off the floor and you find it hard to balance with your hands in Prayer Hands then bring your fingertips to the floor either in front of or behind you or roll up some blankets under your heels.

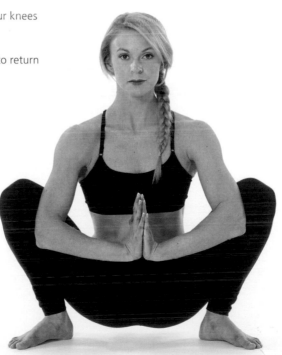

# Toddler Squat

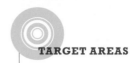

**As children we could squat with our bottom on our heels quite easily, but as adults who sit in chairs most of the day, our mobility decreases and we lose our ability to squat. Toddler Squat helps restore flexibility by encouraging us to adopt a position that is innate.**

**1.** Begin standing with your feet hip-width apart, feet parallel and your toes pointing forwards. Slowly bend your knees to lower your bottom down to your heels.

**2.** Keep your spine long and chest lifted. Focus on relaxing the muscles in your calves and anywhere else you feel restrictions in movement.

**3.** Exit the pose by straightening your legs and returning to standing.

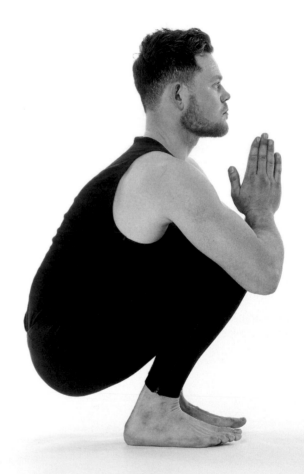

**Variations** -- If you can't squat all the way down then place a rolled up blanket under your heels to increase your range of movement.

**TIPS**

Check in with your feet once you are in the pose to make sure they are parallel.

# Butterfly (yin) & Sleeping Butterfly

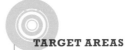

**TARGET AREAS**

**Stretches:** Back, inner thighs
and hamstrings
**Hold Time:** 30–80 breaths

**TIPS**

To target the hamstrings move your feet
further away from you, and to target the
inner thighs draw your heels closer to
your groin

This pose is a passive version of Butterfly (yang) (see
p. 94). Although the name is the same, the intention of
the pose is different. Butterfly (yang) actively stretches
the muscles around the hips whereas Butterfly (yin)
relaxes the muscles and targets the connective tissues
to increase flexibility. Performing a Butterfly (yin) and
Butterfly (yang) back to back increases mobility by
working with the muscles, fascia, connective tissues and
nervous system.

**1.** Begin seated and bring the soles of your feet together with
your heels about foot-distance away from your groin. Fold
forwards, allowing your spine to round. Gently keep hold of your
toes or rest your hands in front of you.

**2.** Focus on relaxing the muscles in your hips and thighs by
visualising your knees sinking closer to the floor.

**3.** Exit the pose by rolling back to seated. Bring your hands to
the outside of your thighs and bring your knees together. Stretch
out your legs in front of you to counter the pose.

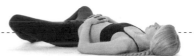

**Variations** -- Sleeping Butterfly is a
lovely alternative to Butterfly (yin). For
this, bring the soles of your feet together
and slowly lower yourself on to your
back. Rest your hands on your belly to
feel yourself breathing or leave them
either side of you with your palms to
the sky.

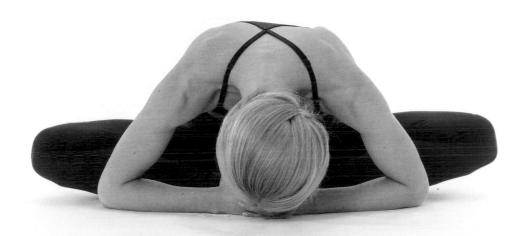

# Half Butterfly (yin)

The yin version of Half Butterfly looks similar to the yang variation (see p. 168). However, instead of lengthening and strengthening the muscles, we are relaxing the muscles and releasing tension from the body with the power of the breath.

**1.** Begin seated in Butterfly (yin) (see p. 167) and straighten your right leg out to the side. Fold forwards by allowing your back to round and rest your hands on the floor in front of you.

**2.** Notice any areas that feel particularly tight and concentrate on relaxing those muscles. Walk your fingers slightly further forwards as your body relaxes.

**3.** Exit the pose by rolling slowly up to seated and repeat with your left leg straight.

**Stretches:** Back, inner thighs and hamstrings
**Hold Time:** 30–50 breaths each side

**TIPS**

Work just outside your comfort zone so you can feel the pose working but you don't feel pain.

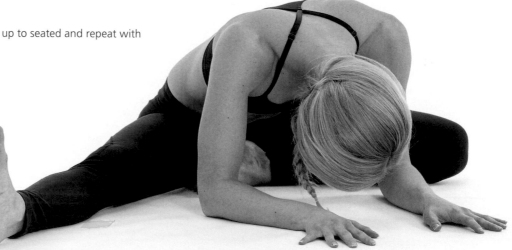

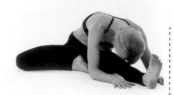

**Variations** -- To target the hamstrings, fold over the outstretched leg.

# Straddle

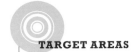

**TARGET AREAS**

**Stretches:** Inner thighs, hamstrings and spine
**Hold Time:** 30–80 breaths

**TIPS**

To get a deeper stretch in the hamstrings, bend the knees so you can get the soles of your feet on the floor, keeping your legs as wide as you can.

We tend to hold a lot of tension in our hips, so Straddle is a great pose to release any tightness. People often find that when they let go of physical tension in poses like Straddle they also feel an emotional release too, so don't be surprised if you feel delicate for a time afterwards.

**1.** Begin seated and spread your legs as wide as you can. Allow your spine to round and fold forwards by walking your fingertips forwards with your weight in your palms.

**2.** Relax here and play your edge by creeping your fingers further forwards as your body opens.

**3.** To exit the pose, push the floor away through your hands and slowly roll up to seated. Bring your legs together and shake them out a little if needed.

**Variations** -- If you feel particularly tight then sit on a cushion or bolster to help tilt your hips forwards.

**Take it up a notch** -- If you can get your chest to the floor then spread your arms out to the sides.

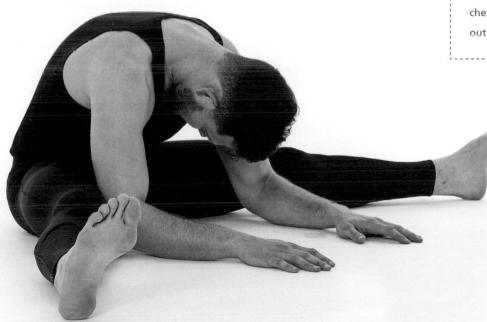

# Sleeping Pigeon

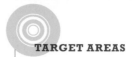

**TARGET AREAS**

**Stretches:** Hips, inner thigh, bottom and lower back

**Hold Time:** 10–30 breaths each side

Sleeping Pigeon opens the hips and releases tension from the lower back. It is a great pose to get to know your body and where you hold your stress. Some people feel a stretch in their inner thigh and others feel it in the outside of the buttock of the bent leg.

**Variations** -- If you feel any pressure in your knee then bring the heel of the bent leg back towards the opposite hip so the shin is diagonal rather than horizontal.

**1.** Begin on all fours in Table Top (see p. 78) and bring your right knee to the outside of your right wrist. Take hold of your right foot and bring your toes to meet your left wrist so your shin is horizontal in front of you. Hook your left toes under and lift your left knee back until you find your edge and feel your hips open. Stay here for a few moments in Pigeon pose to allow gravity to stretch the hips.

**2.** Fold forwards into Sleeping Pigeon by lying your chest on your shin and reaching your arms in front of you. As your muscles relax into the pose, play your edge by sinking your hips closer to the ground and moving your hands further forwards.

**3.** To exit the pose, lift your chest back to Pigeon pose, hook your left toes under and lift yourself back to Table Top or Down Dog (see p. 80). Repeat with the left leg bent in front.

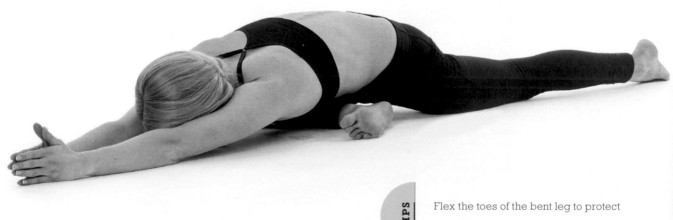

**TIPS**

Flex the toes of the bent leg to protect your knee.

**Keep your hips even to feel the full benefit of the pose.**

# Dragons

**TARGET AREAS**

**Stretches:** Hamstrings and hips
**Hold Time:** 10–30 breaths per Dragon each side

**TIPS**

Notice the difference between pain and discomfort. If you ever feel pain, leave the pose, but if it is slight discomfort then lean into it and allow it to pass.

There are five different styles of Dragon and these can be performed individually or by cycling through all of them to target slightly different areas of the hips and thighs. Each of these poses open the hips deeply, so build up the hold time slowly as your body relaxes and loosens.

**1.** Begin in Table Top (see p. 78) on your hands and knees and step your left foot between your hands so your left knee is directly above the ankle. Slide your right knee back as far as you can, leaving your hands either side of your right foot in Baby Dragon.

**2.** After holding Baby Dragon, move to Dragon Flying High by bringing both hands to rest on your left knee so your torso is upright.

**3.** To work the hips deeper, move to Dragon Flying Low by placing both hands on the inside of your left foot and then moving down on to your forearms.

**4.** Move to Winged Dragon by gently pushing your left knee away from you as you wing out on the outer edge of your foot.

**5.** Move to Twisted Dragon by placing your left hand on your left knee and leaving your right hand on the floor. Twist towards your left knee by rotating your chest to the sky.

**6.** Exit the pose by hooking your right toes under and lifting yourself back to Down Dog (see p. 80) before repeating the Dragons with your left leg forwards.

**Variations --** If your hips are tight and you're feeling pressure in your back knee then roll up a blanket and place it underneath your knee.

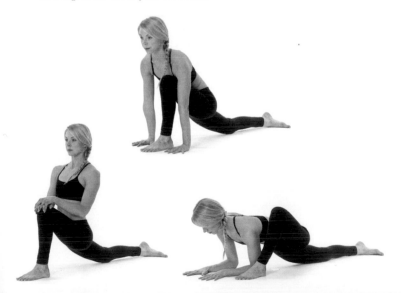

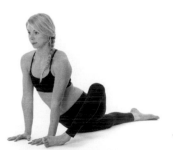

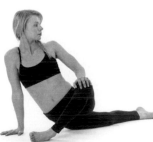

# Shoelace

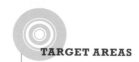

**Stretches:** Hips and lower back
**Hold Time:** 30–50 breaths each side

**Shoelace is a deep hip-opener and a psychologically challenging pose to remain in. If you have been sitting at a desk all day or doing any sport such as cycling for which you are moving your legs up and down rather than side to side or rotating them, then this is a great pose to restore optimum range of movement.**

**1.** Begin sitting cross-legged on the floor and move your right heel to the outside of your left buttock. Stack your left knee on top of your right knee and bring your left heel to the outside of your right buttock.

**2.** Anchor your buttocks to the floor and then bring both feet as far forwards away from your buttocks as you can, keeping your knees stacked. Remain upright or fold forwards and reach your arms out in front of you.

**3.** Exit the pose by rolling back up to seated, leaning back to release the hips and lengthening your legs out in front of you. Repeat with your left knee stacked on top of your right one.

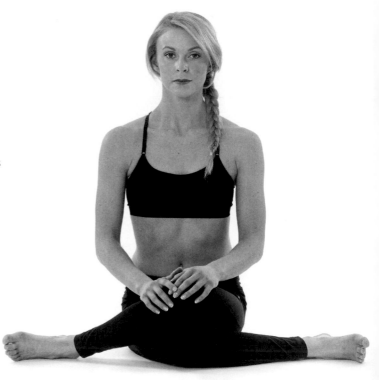

**Variations** -- If it is too challenging to stack your knees on top of each other, then keep the leg that is on top straight in Half Shoelace.

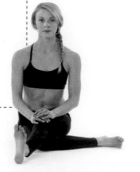

**TIPS**

Visualise the muscles in your hips lengthening and loosening to help you relax into the pose.

# Deer

## TARGET AREAS

**Stretches:** Thighs and hips
**Hold Time:** 30–50 breaths each side

**Deer pose is a deep hip-opener that brings the body into balance through internal and external rotation. You may need to play around with your leg angle and weight distribution until you feel a strong sensation in your hips.**

**1.** Begin seated with the soles of your feet together in Butterfly (yin) pose (see p. 167). Swing your right leg around behind you and position the right foot so your right knee is at a right angle. Move your left foot forwards until your thigh and shin make a right angle.

**2.** When in the pose, focus on rooting both buttocks to the ground. As your hips relax, move your right foot further away from your right hip.

**3.** To exit the pose, lean to the left and bring your right foot back to Butterfly (yin) before repeating with your left leg behind.

**TIPS**

It is easy to tilt away from the back foot so make sure your hips are even and both buttocks are anchored to the ground.

**Notice any difference between the left and right leg and be aware of these throughout your workout or yoga session.**

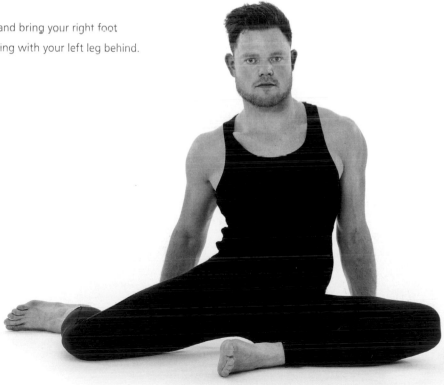

# Sleeping Hero

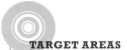

**Stretches:** Thighs, hips and ankles
**Hold Time:** 10–50 breaths

This is a lovely pose to relax in if you've been on your feet all day. Many people, especially runners and cyclists, find the fronts of their thighs can be quite tight, so lower yourself slowly into the pose to give your body an opportunity to get used to the position.

**TIPS**

Keep your back flat to the floor so the pose focuses on the thighs and hips rather than the spine.

If your knees hurt then leave the pose slowly. If you have any existing knee problems, skip this pose.

**1.** Begin kneeling and bring your bottom to the ground in between your feet to Hero pose. Lower yourself backwards on to your elbows and then recline on to your back. Let your arms rest to your side.

**2.** Tune in to any tightness you feel in the fronts of your thighs and your hips and focus on relaxing those muscles so you can sink deeper into the pose.

**3.** Exit the pose the same way as you entered it, by pushing yourself back on to your elbows and up to kneeling. Lift your bottom off the ground before straightening your legs to seated.

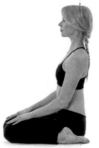

**Variations** -- If you're very tight in your hips or the fronts of your thighs then you may find it challenging to recline in this pose. Instead, remain with your bottom between your heels or sitting on a cushion and your torso upright in Hero. You can also focus on one leg at a time in Half Hero by lengthening one leg out in front of you before you lower yourself on to your back.

**Take it up a notch** -- If you want to deepen the stretch in the front of your thighs then lower yourself into Sleeping Half Hero, for which you bend the outstretched leg and hug the knee towards your chest.

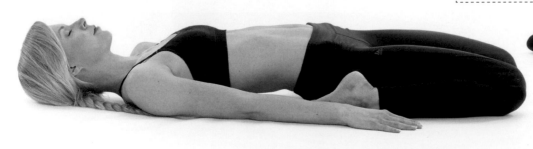

# Frog

**TARGET AREAS**

**Stretches:** Inner thighs and spine
**Hold Time:** 30–50 breaths

**TIPS**

Use padding underneath your knees to protect them if the floor is hard.

Frog is a lovely pose to increase flexibility in your hips. Depending on how open your hips are to begin with, you can start in Tadpole and work your way up to full Frog as your body learns the posture and relaxes into it.

**1.** Begin in Child's Pose (see p. 180) and reach forwards with your arms to bring your palms to the ground. Spread your knees as wide as you can into Tadpole, then separate your feet so they are in line with your knees and your shins are parallel.

**2.** Give yourself enough time in this pose for your hips and thighs to release to allow you to fully relax.

**3.** Exit the pose by bringing your toes and knees together and shift your bottom back to Child's Pose.

**Variations** -- If your hips are tight then leave your toes together in Tadpole or lift your hips to bring them in line with your knees in Half Frog so gravity can have more impact on the pose.

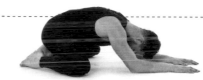

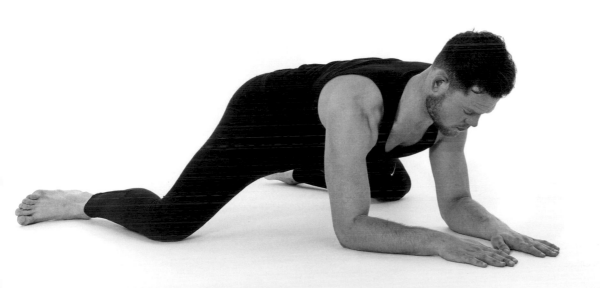

# Neck Release

**Stretches:** Neck and shoulders

**Hold Time:** 10 breaths each side

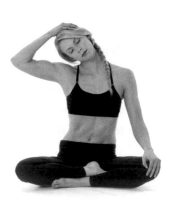

**We hold a lot of tension in our neck and shoulders from looking at computer screens, driving and other activities of daily living. Tight neck muscles are a common cause of headaches and migraines and can also affect your breathing so it is important to keep the neck mobile.**

**1.** Begin in any comfortable seated position. Begin with lateral flexion of the neck by dropping your right ear towards your right shoulder. Bring your right hand to rest on the side of your head to increase the stretch. Release and repeat to the left.

**2.** For forward flexion of the neck, lengthen the top of your head to the sky as you inhale and then as you exhale stick your chin forwards and bring your chin towards your chest. Interlace your fingers and rest your palms on the back of your head with your elbows hanging down towards the floor. Release the pose by taking your hands off the back of your head and slowly rolling your head back up to neutral.

**3.** For neck extension, lengthen the crown of your head to the sky as you inhale and drop your head back slowly as you exhale. Open your mouth if you need to and notice any sensations. Come out of the pose by bringing your head back to neutral.

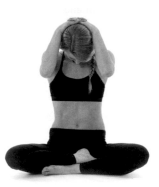

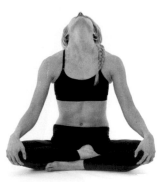

**TIPS**

When resting your hand on your head, don't push down but allow the weight of gravity to increase the stretch.

# Melting Heart

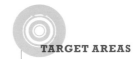

## TARGET AREAS

**Stretches:** Back and shoulders
**Hold Time:** 30–50 breaths

**Melting Heart is a gentle backbend that can be used as a warm-up before deeper yang backbends such as Camel (see p. 108) and Bridge (see p. 107). We tend to hold a lot of tension in our spine and shoulders so it is also a wonderful pose to do after a long day at work to help you release any stress and calm any anxiety.**

**TIPS**

If you feel any pinching in your shoulders then move your hands a bit further apart.

As any tightness in your shoulders and upper back subsides and your body opens, move into that space by walking your fingers slightly further forwards.

**1.** Begin on all fours in Table Top (see p. 78) and walk your fingers forwards. Allow your chest to sink towards the floor and rest your forehead on the ground. Aim to keep your hips stacked over your knees and your hands shoulder-width apart.

**2.** Focus on releasing any tightness from the shoulders and upper back. Channel every inhale into any areas of tension and with each exhale allow yourself to soften deeper into the pose as your muscles relax.

**3.** To come out of the pose, slowly shift your bottom to your heels and wrap your arms around behind you with your palms to the sky. Rest here in Child's Pose (see p. 180) for a moment before pushing back to Table Top.

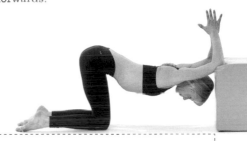

**Take it up a notch --** To target the shoulders more deeply, come into Table Top in front of a stable surface and rest your upper arms on the edge of the surface. Bend your elbows and bring your palms together so your fingertips are facing the ceiling and sink your head down between your arms.

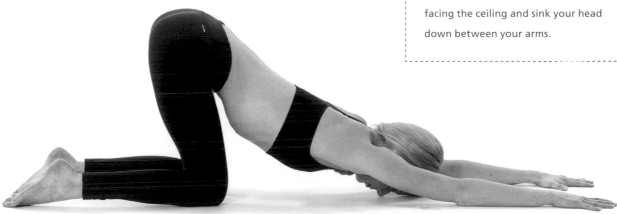

# Caterpillar

**Relaxes:** Back, neck and hamstrings
**Hold Time:** 30–50 breaths

**Caterpillar is a relaxing forward bend. Unlike yang forward bends, for which the aim is to keep the spine long, in yin forward bends you allow the spine to round and the head to hang. This positively stresses the ligaments in the spine to strengthen them and releases tension in the back and hamstrings to increase flexibility.**

**1.** Begin seated with both legs lengthened out in front of you. Fold forwards, allowing your back to round and resting your forehead on your shins or letting your head hang. Rest your arms either side of your legs.

**2.** Give your body the time and space to relax in this pose without any pushing or pulling. As you feel your muscles loosen then move into the slack that's created to deepen the pose.

**3.** To exit the pose, slowly roll up to seated.

**TIPS**

Feel free to bend your knees slightly if it makes the pose more comfortable.

Notice whether restrictions in movement are coming from the backs of your legs or your lower back and focus on relaxing those muscles.

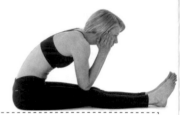

**Variations** -- If you feel tension in your neck then place a cushion on your legs to rest your head on, or bend your arms and rest your head in your hands.

**Take it up a notch** -- See if you can spread your legs slightly and allow your chest to sink down in between them.

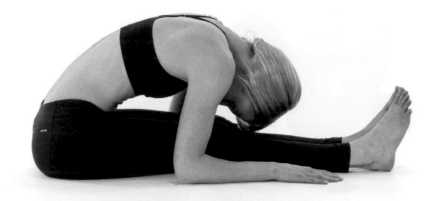

# Baby Cobra (yin)

**TARGET AREAS**

**Relaxes:** Lower back and belly
**Hold Time:** 10–50 breaths

**TIPS**

This is a great pose to watch television in instead of slumping on the sofa.

**Baby Cobra (yin) is a baby backbend that is held very passively. Unlike the yang version, you are not attempting to strengthen your shoulders; instead you are focusing on the healthy compression in your lower back, which is very therapeutic and energising.**

**1.** Begin lying on your belly and bring your forearms to the floor with your hands just in front of your shoulders. Lift your chest to prop yourself up on your forearms.

**2.** Allow your shoulders to relax in the pose and let your head hang back to stretch out the front of the neck if that feels good.

**3.** To exit the pose, slowly lower your chest to the floor and counter pose with a gentle forward bend such as Caterpillar (see p. 182).

**Variations** -- If the sensation in your back is too strong then slide your forearms forwards to lower your chest closer to the floor.

**Take it up a notch** -- If you have a healthy spine then you can deepen the back bend to Up Dog (see p. 102). Bring your hands either side of your chest and straighten your arms to lift your chest.

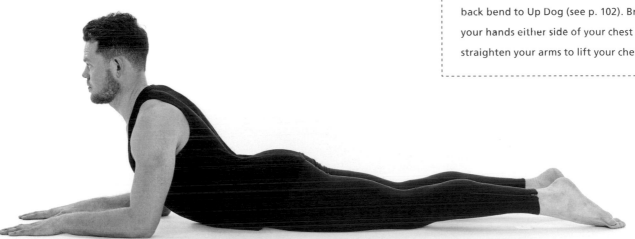

# Sleeping Crocodile

## TARGET AREAS

**Relaxes:** Spine, hips and neck

**Hold Time:** 10–30 breaths

TIPS

Do Sleeping Crocodile in between backbends such as Baby Cobra (yin) (see p. 183) as a counter pose.

**This is a great counter pose to any backbends and releases any tension from the spine. The more relaxed you are, the higher you will be able to get your knee and the greater the release you will feel.**

**1.** Begin lying on your belly with your arms bent and palms resting on the floor by your head. Turn your head to the right and draw your right knee up beside you on the floor.

**2.** Focus on relaxing your inner thigh as well as letting go of any tension in your spine.

**3.** To exit the pose, straighten your leg and return your head to centre before repeating to the left side.

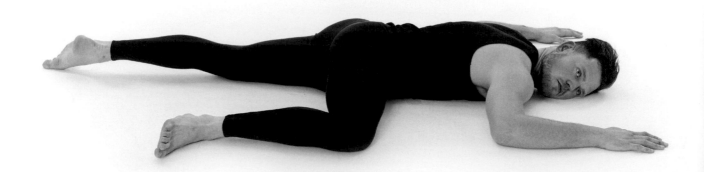

# Banana

**Relaxes:** Waist, hips and spine

**Hold Time:** 30–50 breaths each side

Visualise the muscles down your side lengthening so you can deepen the bend of your Banana.

**To increase the stretch, cross your ankles once you are in your Banana.**

Banana stretches the entire side of the body. We usually only move our spine forwards and backwards so by bending the spine laterally you release tension and increase mobility. The more flexible your spine, the more bendy your Banana will be.

**1.** Begin lying on your back with your legs together. Reach your arms over your head and take hold of each elbow. Keeping your bottom on the ground, move your feet as far as you can to the left and then move your upper body as far as you can to the left.

**2.** Find your edge so that you feel a gentle opening down your right-hand side, from your armpit all the way past your ribcage and waist and into the outside of your hips. As your spine opens move your feet and upper body further to the left.

**3.** Come back to centre to release the pose and then bend your Banana to the right.

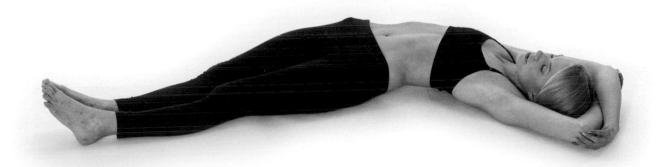

# Reclining Twist

Adjust the height of your leg to target a specific area of the spine. The higher you have your knees, the higher you will feel the twist in your spine.

**Passive twists are perfect for the end of your Yoga Gym workout or yoga session to allow the body to fully relax and release. As well as releasing tension from the spine, they rebalance the nervous system and massage the internal organs to help detoxify the body.**

**1.** Begin lying on your back and hug your left knee into your chest. Take hold of the outside of your left knee with your right hand and bring your left leg across your body. Keep both shoulder blades on the floor and look over your left shoulder.

**2.** Either keep your left leg bent or see if you can straighten it and take hold of your left big toe with your right forefingers to increase the twist.

**3.** Come out of the pose by releasing your toe or knee, rolling on to your back and hugging your knees into your chest. Repeat with your right leg.

**Variations** -- For a simple twist, hug your knees into your chest and then let both knees fall across to your right as you turn to look over your left shoulder. Repeat with your knees to the left while looking over your right shoulder.

# Legs Up The Wall

## TARGET AREAS

**Relaxes:** Lower back and hamstrings
**Hold Time:** 30–80 breaths

**TIPS**

Incorporate some breathing exercises when doing this pose to help you relax.

Inversions are very restorative. They bring the blood back to the heart and lungs and relax the nervous system. Legs Up The Wall pose allows you to completely relax at the same time as lengthening your hamstrings and releasing any tension from your lower back. If you have had a long day and don't fancy a full Yoga Gym workout then use the time to rest and restore in this pose.

**1.** Sit sideways against the wall and swing your legs around so you are lying on your back with your Legs Up The Wall. Bring your bottom as close the wall as you can and straighten your legs, resting your heels on the wall. Spread your arms out sideways.

**2.** Rest here for as long as you need to. Focus on relaxing any areas of tension in your body.

**3.** To exit the pose, move your bottom away from the wall slightly and swivel your legs down to one side before pushing up to seated.

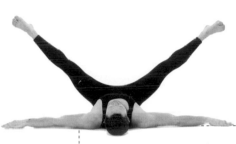

> **Variations** -- You can bring your feet together in Butterfly (yin) pose (see p. 167), move your legs into a wide squat or spread them wide in Straddle (see p. 169) for some alternative wall postures.

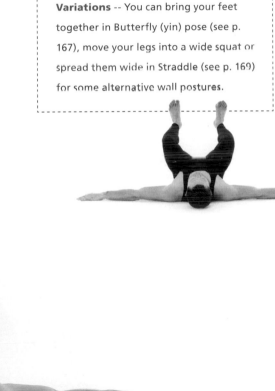

# Shoulder Stand

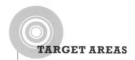

**Shoulder Stand takes elements from both yin and yang postures. It requires muscular effort to maintain alignment, which strengthens and stretches the body and also encourages the nervous system to relax to leave you feeling re-energised.**

**1.** Lie on your back and bring your legs up and over your head. Place your hands on your lower back with your fingers facing your bottom, engage your core and bring your legs up to vertical so your toes are pointing towards the sky.

**2.** Aim to bring your ankles over your knees, your knees over your hips and your hips over your shoulders. Be sure to have most of your weight in your upper arms and shoulders with minimal weight in your neck.

**3.** Exit the pose by slowly rolling back down to the floor.

**Variations** -- If you feel any discomfort in your neck then Legs Up The Wall pose (see p. 187) is a good alternative.

**TIPS**

Squeeze your buttocks to help keep your pelvis stable and spine in alignment.

Draw your elbows closer together and push your upper arms into the ground to open your chest.

# Plough

TARGET AREAS

**Relaxes:** Spine and neck

**Hold Time:** 30–50 breaths

Plough is also known as Snail pose and is a lovely pose to perform at the end of a Yoga Gym workout or yoga session. It releases the spine and relaxes the whole **posterior kinetic chain** – a series of muscles in the back of the body. Because it is an inversion it also calms the nervous system to leave you feeling centred and refreshed.

**TIPS**

Position most of the weight of your body in your shoulders with very little weight in your neck.

**Prepare for the pose by doing the Neck Release stretches (see p.178)**

1. Begin lying on your back and lift your legs up and over your head so your toes are on the floor. Interlace your fingers and allow your arms to rest on the floor in front of you.

2. Allow the spine to round, keeping your neck long so you can still breathe deeply.

3. To exit the pose, bring your hands to your lower back, bend your knees and lower yourself back down slowly to the ground. Rest here for a couple of moments to allow your blood pressure to readjust before sitting up.

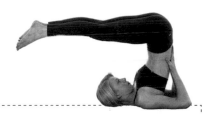

**Variations** -- If your toes don't touch the ground, you can either keep your legs parallel to the floor or bend your knees and rest them on your forehead.

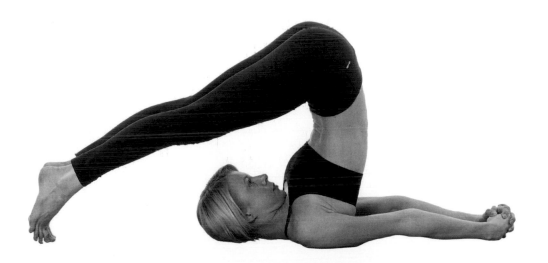

# Seagull Arms

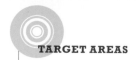

**Wrist problems are common in people who type and drive a lot, so Seagull Arms is a great stretch to strengthen the tissues in the wrists. People who are new to yoga often find they get wrist pain in positions such as Down Dog (see p. 80) and Plank (see p. 84), and Seagull Arms works well as a counter pose.**

**1.** Sit or stand in any comfortable position. Snuggle the back of your hands underneath your armpits with your elbows winging out to the side.

**2.** As your wrists begin to relax then slowly lower your elbows closely to your body to deepen the pose.

**3.** Exit the pose by releasing your hands by your sides and wiggling your fingers.

**Variations** -- You can also massage out your wrists by bringing the backs of your hands together or by performing Table Top (see p. 78) and bringing the back of your hands to rest on the floor one at a time.

**TIPS**

Use this pose in between arm balances, such as Plank (see p. 84), Crocodile (see p. 88) and Crow (see p. 87), to help refresh your wrists.

# Cow Face Arms

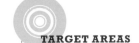

**This is one of the best poses for loosening up your shoulders. You can add in Cow Face Arms to many seated postures such as Butterfly (yin) (see p. 167), Lotus (see p. 100), and Hero (see p. 174) to relax and stretch your hips and arms simultaneously.**

**1.** Begin in any seated or standing position. Reach your left hand to the sky and bend your arm behind your head to pat yourself on the back. Bring your right arm down and behind your back and reach your right fingertips up as high as you can between your shoulder blades to take hold of your left hand.

**2.** Find your edge and lean into any discomfort to allow your shoulders to loosen and open.

**3.** Release your hands and stretch your arms out to the side to open your shoulders even more. Allow your arms to rest beside you before repeating with the right arm over the left arm below.

**TARGET AREAS**

**Relaxes:** Shoulders
**Hold Time:** 1–3 minutes each side

**TIPS**

Keep your shoulders relaxed away from your ears to allow your upper body to fully release.

Bring your top elbow as far across to the centre of the head as you can so you can reach your fingers further down your back.

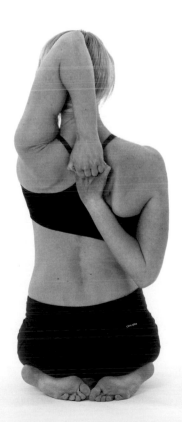

**Variations** -- If you can't take hold of your hands then use a strap or belt to grasp on to.

# Reverse Prayer

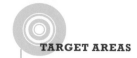

**Relaxes:** Shoulders and chest
**Hold Time:** 10–30 breaths

**If you spend a lot of time hunched over a desk then Reverse Prayer is a great pose to do throughout the day to release stress from your shoulders and realign your spine.**

**1.** Sit or stand in a comfortable position and reach your hands behind you so the backs of your hands are flat between your shoulder blades with your little fingers touching. Let your shoulders fall forwards as you bring your palms together. Roll your shoulders back and down to open your chest.

**2.** Work at your edge by pulling your elbows back to keep your chest open.

**3.** Release the pose slowly by reaching your arms out to the side with your palms facing forwards.

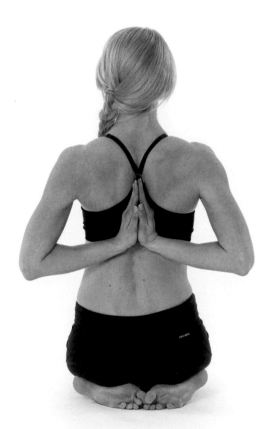

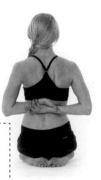

**Variations** -- If you can't get your palms together then bring the backs of your hands together or take hold of the opposite wrist behind your back.

**TIPS**

Do this pose several times a day to stop you from storing stress in your shoulders and prevent tension headaches.

# Corpse

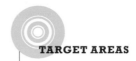

**Relaxes:** Full body
**Hold Time:** As long as possible

This is the easiest but also the most difficult pose of them all. In the hectic world we live in, relaxation is greatly undervalued and we can even feel guilty for allowing ourselves to relax. Corpse pose forces us to stop and give our body and mind the opportunity to absorb our workout or yoga practice and fully relax.

**1.** Lie down on your back and begin by taking a deep inhalation, stretching your arms above your head, pointing your toes and engaging every muscle in your body. As you exhale, release all the tension from your body, bring your arms down by your sides with your palms to the sky and allow your feet to wing out just wider than hip-width apart. If you have any back pain then you can also bend your knees and let them fall inwards.

**2.** Release any control over your breathing and allow every muscle in your body to completely relax. Stay here for as long as you want.

**3.** When you are ready to come out of the pose, start by wiggling your fingers and toes and then circle your ankles and your wrists. Hug your knees into your chest or have a stretch and a yawn and then roll over on to your right side. Spend a couple of moments here to rebalance your blood pressure before pushing yourself up slowly to a comfortable seated position.

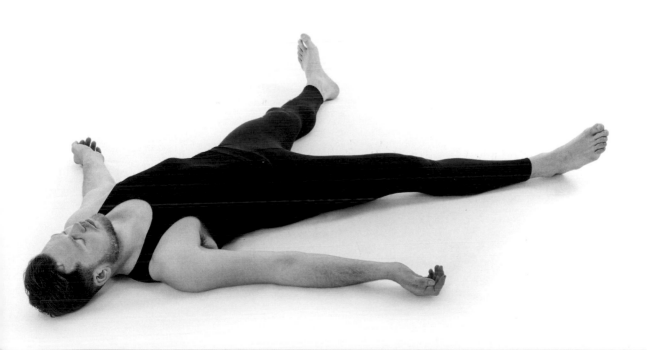

# Challenge poses

If you want more of a challenge there are many more advanced yoga poses to have a go at, including those below. These are beyond the scope of this book but you can find detailed instructions at www.YogaGymRevolution.com.

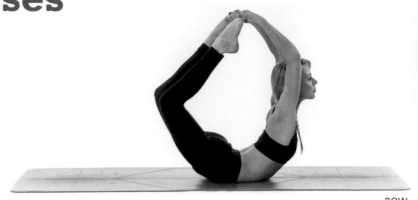

BOW

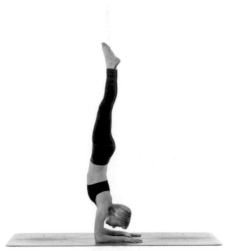

FOREARM STAND

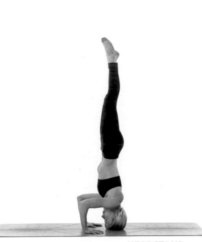

HEADSTAND

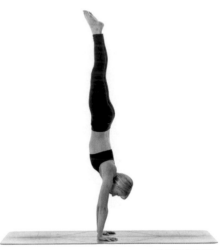

HANDSTAND

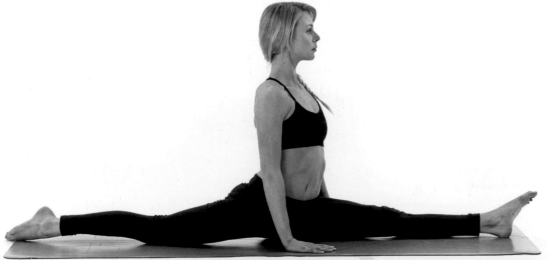

SPLITS

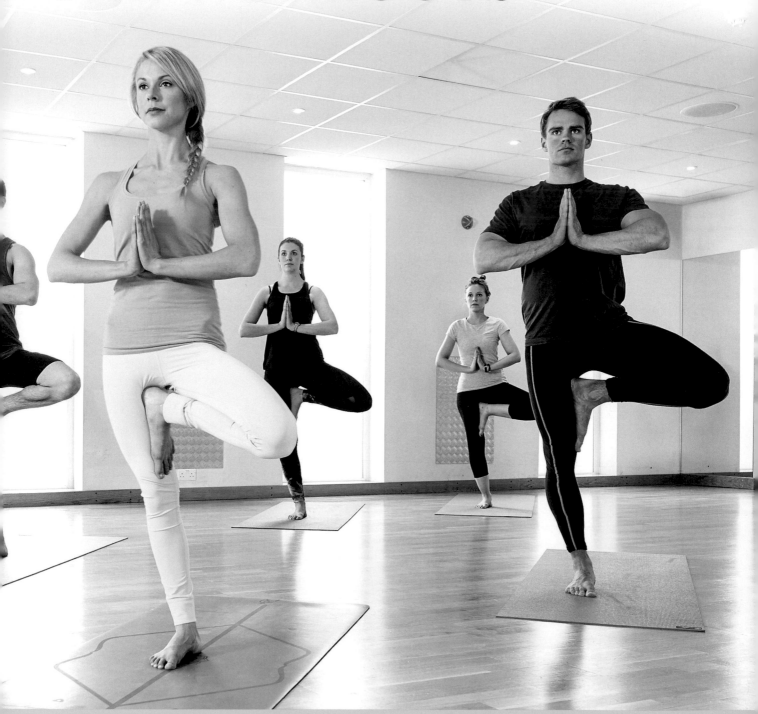

# PART 3
# THE WORKOUTS

# Using the Yoga Gym plan

**The 28-day Yoga Gym plan is aimed to ignite your passion for yoga and bodyweight training and set you on the path to strength, flexibility and fat loss. It is not a one-month miracle plan (any product claiming to be a one-stop quick-fix is lying) but it is designed to get maximum results in as little time as possible.**

The plan is made up of five workouts a week. Each workout lasts between 30–50 minutes and is suitable for all abilities – just pick the yoga pose and yogacise variations that suit your fitness level from Part 2 of the book. Once you've completed the plan, you can take a few days off and begin again using more challenging versions of each pose and yogacise. As your fitness level improves you can keep adapting the 28-day plan by including harder variations of each pose and yogacise so you keep getting stronger, leaner and more flexible.

The plan uses periodisation to get the greatest strength and flexibility gains at the same time as preventing over-training and risk of injury. Different intensities are used across the weeks, as well as various numbers of repetitions and sets and differing lengths of rest periods. Changing the volume and intensity of the workouts will keep your body guessing, your metabolism fast and your motivation high.

If your motivation does dwindle at any point then you can find some motivational videos on my website www.YogaGymRevolution.com. There is also a 28-day calendar at www.bloomsbury.com/9781472912886 for you to download so you can schedule in your workout sessions.

# How the workouts work

Each workout is a sequence of breathing exercises, yang poses, yogacises and yin poses.

This sequence begins with the most basic form of movement – breathing, followed by the dynamic element of the workout (flows, yang poses and yogacises) including a finisher yogacise that will test how many push-ups, squats or crunches you can do. Recording the number of repetitions you do in your finisher yogacise is a good way to track your progress. Each workout ends with a few minutes of relaxing yin yoga to allow the body and mind to absorb the full benefits of the session.

# Types of workout

There are five types of workout in the Yoga Gym plan. Each type emphasises different areas of fitness to build strength, power and cardiovascular fitness, as well as increasing flexibility, burning fat and encouraging relaxation.

The workouts are divided into upper body, lower body, core, and full-body workouts, with the type of workout varying each week.

Week 1 workouts have an emphasis on strength by using interval training. In week 2, the focus shifts to building power through supersets. Week 3 uses high-intensity training known as Tabatas to ignite fat loss. And week 4 varies the type of workout each session to really challenge you. Each week you will also perform a Body Blast workout combining resistance and cardiovascular exercise using PHA Training where you complete an upper body exercise immediately followed by a lower body exercise, and a yin workout to restore optimal mobility and rebalance the nervous system. The yin workout is different from all other workouts in that it consists purely of breathing exercises and yin poses.

Although it may not seem as calorie-burning or muscle-building as the other workouts, it is essential you do the full yin workout each week to help your body recover from the more active sessions.

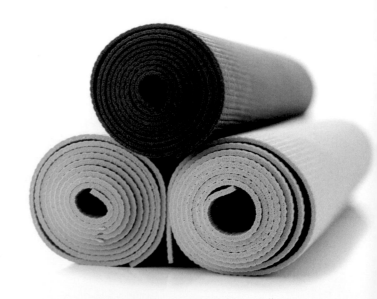

The types of workouts are described in more detail below:

## INTERVAL

**Benefits:** Increased strength, fat loss, improved body awareness

- 3 sets per yogacise
- 12 repetitions per set
- 60 seconds' rest after each set
- If you can't reach 12 repetitions then 'work to failure', i.e. until you can no longer do any more, for each yogacise
- For all single-leg yogacises, do all repetitions on your non-dominant, or weaker, leg before repeating on your dominant, or stronger, leg immediately afterwards

## SUPERSET

**Benefits:** Increased strength and power, increased muscle mass, fat loss, time efficient

- 3 supersets per yogacise pair
- Perform stated repetitions for the first yogacise in each pair and then immediately follow with the second yogacise in the pair with no rest
- 30–60 seconds' rest in between each superset
- For single-legged yogacises, alternate sides after each repetition

## TABATA

**Benefits:** Fat loss, increased metabolic rate, improved cardiovascular fitness, quick and efficient

- 5 yogacises per Tabata circuit
- 20 seconds per yogacise, then 10 seconds' rest before moving on to the next yogacise
- 4 rounds per circuit
- For single-legged yogacises, alternate sides after each rep
- This is high-intensity training

## PERIPHERAL HEART ACTION (PHA) TRAINING

**Benefits:** Increased strength, improved cardiovascular fitness, fat loss, reduced lactic acid build-up so faster recovery

- 8–10 yogacises per circuit
- 5–10 repetitions per yogacise
- Complete as many rounds of the circuit as possible in 20 minutes
- For single-legged yogacises, alternate sides after each
- This combines resistance and aerobic training by getting you to perform an upper-body yogacise followed by a lower-body yogacise

## YIN

**Benefits:** Increased flexibility and range of movement, quicker recovery times between workouts, reduced stress, improved focus

- Recovery session
- 10–20 yin poses per workout
- Ends with a 10-minute relaxation

# Warm-ups

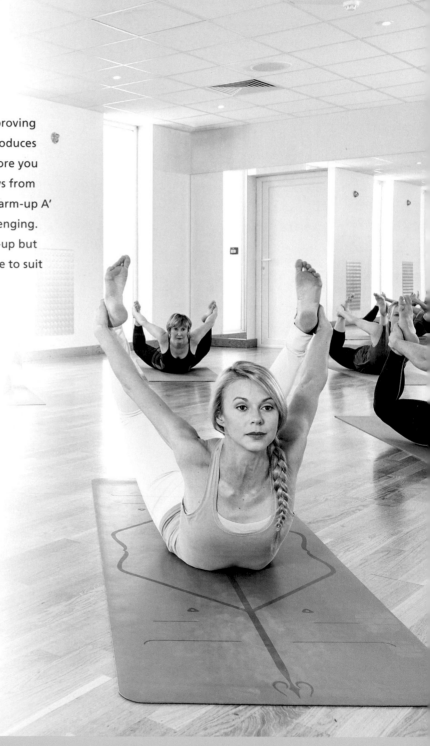

Warming up the body properly is crucial for improving strength and flexibility. The Yoga Gym plan introduces you to four warm-up sequences to perform before you work out. These consist of combinations of flows from Part 2 of the book and increase in difficulty: 'Warm-up A' is the easiest and 'Warm-up D' is the most challenging. Each Yoga Gym workout has a suggested warm-up but you can select a gentler or more challenging one to suit your fitness and energy level.

**WARM-UP A**
5 (each side) x Eagle Flow (see p. 112)
2 x Y Flow (see p. 115)
3 x Sun Salutation A (see p. 116)

**WARM-UP B**
1 minute x Cat and Cow (see p. 111)
1 minute x Forward Bend Flow (see p. 114)
3 x Sun Salutation A (see p. 116)

**WARM-UP C**
3 x Sun Salutation A (see p. 116)
2 x Sun Salutation B (see p. 118)

**WARM-UP D**
5 x Sun Salutation A (see p. 116)
3 x Sun Salutation B (see p. 118)

# Weekly session plans

**WEEK 1**

**SESSION 1**

**Focus:** Upper body

**Training type:** Intervals

---

**5 ROUNDS**

Four Face Breathing (see p. 54)

---

**Warm Up A** (see p. 200)

---

**2 ROUNDS**

5 breaths x Mountain (see p. 59)

5 breaths x Down Dog (see p. 80)

5 breaths x Dolphin (see p. 82)

5 breaths x Plank (see p. 84)

5 breaths x Crocodile (see p. 88)

*Place your hips on the floor or on a block if required.*

5 breaths x Baby Cobra (yang) (see p. 101)

OR Up Dog (see p. 102)

---

**3 ROUNDS**

12 x Down Dog Push-ups (see p. 127)

Rest @ 60 seconds

---

**3 ROUNDS**

12 x Narrow Push-ups (see p. 123)

*Push off a wall or elevate your hands on a surface if you need to.*

Rest @ 60 seconds

---

**3 ROUNDS**

12 x Rocking Planks (see p. 129)

Rest @ 60 seconds

---

**3 ROUNDS**

12 x Reverse Table Top Dips (see p. 130)

Raise your hands on a surface if required.

Rest @ 60 seconds

---

**1 ROUND**

Maximum number of Classic Push-ups

(see p. 122) in 1 minute

*Push off a wall or elevate your hands on a surface if you need to.*

---

**1 ROUND**

20 breaths x Melting Heart (see p. 179)

10 breaths x Child's Pose (see p. 180)

10 breaths each side x Thread The Needle (see p. 181)

30 breaths x Legs Up The Wall (see p. 187)

---

WORK TO FAILURE IF YOU CAN'T REACH
12 REPETITIONS FOR EACH EXERCISE.

**WEEK 1**

**WORKOUT 2**

**Focus:** Lower body

**Training type:** Intervals

---

**1 ROUND**

10 rounds x Three Part Breath (see p. 55)

---

# Warm-up B (see p. 200)

---

**1 ROUND**

10 breaths x Baby Bridge (see p. 106)

10 breaths x Chair (see p. 62)

10 breaths x Standing Forward Bend (see p. 65)

5 breaths x Triangle (right) (see p. 68)

5 breaths x Side Angle (right) (see p. 70)

5 breaths x Triangle (left)

5 breaths x Side Angle (left)

10 breaths x Standing Wide Leg Forward Bend (see p. 67)

10 breaths x Sun God (see p. 63)

---

**3 ROUNDS**

12 x Sumo Squats (see p. 136) with 3-seconds
pause at bottom

Rest @ 60 seconds

---

**3 ROUNDS**

12 x Glute Bridges (see p. 147) with 3-second hold at top

Rest @ 60 seconds

---

**3 ROUNDS**

12 each side x Split Squats (see p. 143)

Rest @ 60 seconds

---

**3 ROUNDS**

12 each side x Side Lunges (see p. 144)

Rest @ 60 seconds

---

**1 ROUND**

Maximum number of Squats (see p. 135) in 1 minute

---

**1 ROUND**

10 breaths x Ragdoll (see p. 164)

20 breaths x Wide Squat (see p. 165)

20 breaths each side x Sleeping Pigeon (see p. 170)

---

WORK TO FAILURE IF YOU CAN'T REACH
12 REPETITIONS FOR EACH EXERCISE.

**Focus:** Core

**Training type:** Intervals

**3 ROUNDS**

Stomach Pumping Breath (see p. 57)

# Warm-up C (see p. 200)

**1 ROUND**

10 breaths x Plank (see p. 84)

5 breaths x Boat (see p. 89)

10 breaths x Plank

5 breaths per leg x Tree (see p. 76)

10 breaths x Plank

5 breaths x Locust (see p. 105)

10 breaths each side x Seated Twist (see p. 92)

**3 ROUNDS**

12 x Hinges (see p. 151)

Rest @ 60 seconds

**3 ROUNDS**

12 x Half Moon Bends (see p. 152)

Rest @ 60 seconds

**3 ROUNDS**

12 x Locust Lifts (see p. 157)

Rest @ 60 seconds

**3 ROUNDS**

12 x Iron Crosses (see p. 153)

Rest @ 60 seconds

**1 ROUND**

Maximum number of Crunches (see p. 159) in 1 minute

**1 ROUND**

20 breaths x Baby Cobra (yang) (see p. 101)

OR Up Dog (see p. 102)

10 breaths each side x Banana (see p. 184)

10 breaths each side x Reclining Twist (see p. 186)

10 breaths x Shoulder stand (see p. 188)

OR Legs Up The Wall (see p. 187)

WORK TO FAILURE IF YOU CAN'T REACH
12 REPETITIONS FOR EACH EXERCISE.

---

**1 ROUND**

2 minutes x Ocean Breath (see p. 53)

---

# Warm-up B (see p. 200)

---

**1 ROUND**

10 breaths x Chair (see p. 62)

10 breaths each side x Twisted Chair (see p. 64)

10 breaths x Standing Forward Bend (see p. 65)

10 breaths x Warrior 2 (right) (see p. 73)

10 breaths x Warrior 1 (right) (see p. 72)

10 breaths x Warrior 3 (right) (see p. 74)

10 breaths x Warrior 2 (left)

10 breaths x Warrior 1 (left)

10 breaths x Warrior 3 (left)

---

*Complete this circuit as many times
as you can in 20 minutes:*

5 x Classic Push-ups (see p.122)

10 x Squats (see p. 135)

5 x Down Dog Push-ups (see p. 127)

10 x Sumo Squats (see p. 136)

5 x Reverse Table Top Dips (see p. 130)

10 each side x Split Squats (see p. 143)

5 x Narrow Push-ups (see p. 123)

10 x Iron Crosses (see p. 153)

---

**1 ROUND**

20 breaths x Caterpillar (see p. 182)

20 breaths x Butterfly  (see p. 167)

20 breaths x Sleeping Butterfly (see p. 167)

---

**10 ROUNDS**

Square Breathing (see p. 56)

---

**1 ROUND**

10 breaths each side x Neck Release (see p. 178)

20 breaths x Butterfly (yin) (see p. 167)

10 breaths x Windshield Wipers (see p. 113)

10 breaths x Half Butterfly (yin) (right) (see p. 168)

10 breaths x Windshield Wipers

10 breaths x Half Butterfly (yin) (left)

10 breaths x Windshield Wipers

10 breaths x Child's Pose (see p. 180)

20 breaths x Melting Heart (see p. 179)

10 breaths x Child's Pose

20 breaths x Dragons (right) (see p. 171)

10 breaths x Rocking Table Top (see p. 120)

20 breaths x Dragons (left) (see p. 171)

10 breaths x Rocking Table Top

20 breaths each side x Half Shoelace (see p. 172)

20 breaths x Happy Baby (see p. 177)

30 breaths x Legs Up The Wall (see p. 189)

100 breaths x Corpse (see p. 193)

**Focus:** Upper body

**Training type:** Supersets

---

**3 ROUNDS**

Four Face Breathing (see p. 54)

---

# Warm-up A (see p. 200)

---

**2 ROUNDS**

10 breaths x Down Dog (see p. 80)

10 breaths each side x Three-legged Dog (see p. 81)

10 breaths each side x One-legged Plank (see p. 84)

10 breaths x Up Dog (see p. 102)

---

**3 ROUNDS**

6 x Yoga Push-ups (see p. 124)

12 x Down Dog Push-ups (see p. 127)

*Push off a wall or elevate your hands on a surface if you need to.*

Rest @ 30–60 seconds

---

**3 ROUNDS**

6 x Windmill Push-ups (see p. 128)

12 x Narrow Push-ups (see p. 123)

*Push off a wall or elevate your hands on a surface if you need to.*

Rest @ 30–60 seconds

---

**3 ROUNDS**

6 x Crocodile Push-ups (see p. 125)

12 x Rocking Plank (see p. 129)

*Push off a wall or elevate your hands on a surface if you need to.*

Rest @ 30–60 seconds

---

**1 ROUND**

Maximum number of Classic Push-ups (see p. 122) in 1 minute

*Push off a wall or elevate your hands on a surface if you need to.*

---

**1 ROUND**

20 breaths x Melting Heart (see p. 179)

20 breaths each side x Thread The Needle (see p. 181)

20 breaths x Plough (see p. 189)

**Focus:** Lower body

**Training type:** Supersets

**1 ROUND**

10 breaths x Three Part Breath (see p. 55)

# Warm-up B (see p. 200)

**1 ROUND**

10 breaths x Baby Bridge (see p. 106)

10 breaths x Chair (see p. 62)

10 breaths x Standing Forward Bend (see p. 65)

10 breaths x Side Angle (right) (see p. 70)

10 breaths x Warrior 2 (right) (see p. 73)

10 breaths x Warrior 1 (right) (see p. 72)

10 x Warrior 3 (right) (see p. 74)

10 breaths x Side Angle (left)

10 breaths x Warrior 2 (left)

10 breaths x Warrior 1 (left)

10 x Warrior 3 (left)

**3 ROUNDS**

6 each side x One-legged Squats (see p. 137)

12 x Squat Jumps (see p. 138)

Rest @ 30–60 seconds

**3 ROUNDS**

6 each side x Lunge (see p. 140) with 3-second pause at bottom

12 x Mountain Climbers (see p. 145)

Rest @ 30–60 seconds

**3 ROUNDS**

6 each side x Warrior Lifts (see p. 146)

12 x Star Jumps (see p. 139)

Rest @ 30–60 seconds

**1 ROUND**

Maximum number of Squats (see p. 135) in 1 minute

**1 ROUND**

20 breaths x Ragdoll (see p. 164)

20 breaths x Wide Squat (see p. 165)

20 breaths each side x Sleeping Pigeon (see p. 170)

**WEEK 2**

**SESSION 3**

**Focus:** Core

**Training type:** Supersets

---

**3 ROUNDS**

Stomach Pumping Breath (see p. 57)

---

**Warm-up C** (see p. 200)

---

**1 ROUND**

20 breaths x Plank (see p. 84)

10 breaths each side x Three-legged Dog (see p. 87)

20 breaths x Plank

10 breaths x Locust (see p. 105)

20 breaths x Plank

10 breaths x Reverse Table Top (see p. 103)

---

**3 ROUNDS**

6 x Rocking Boats (see p. 154)

12 x Flutter Kicks (see p. 160)

Rest @ 30–60 seconds

---

**3 ROUNDS**

6 x Hip-ups (see p. 156)

12 x Locust Lifts (see p. 157)

Rest @ 30–60 seconds

---

**3 ROUNDS**

6 each side x Triple Down Dogs (see p. 155)

12 x Yogic Bicycles (see p. 158)

Rest @ 30–60 seconds

---

**1 ROUND**

Maximum number of Crunches (see p. 159) in 1 minute

---

**1 ROUND**

20 breaths x Baby Cobra (yin) (see p. 183)

10 breaths each side x Sleeping Crocodile (see p. 184)

10 breaths x Camel (see p. 108)

10 breaths each side x Banana (see p. 184)

10 breaths each side x Reclining Twist (see p. 186)

**1 ROUND**

2 minutes x Ocean Breath (see p. 53)

**Warm-up C** (see p. 200)

**1 ROUND**

10 breaths x Bear (see p. 79)

10 breaths x Warrior 2 (right) (see p. 73)

10 breaths x Warrior 1 (right) (see p. 72)

10 breaths x Warrior 3 (right) (see p. 74)

10 breaths x Warrior 2 (left)

10 breaths x Warrior 1 (left)

10 breaths x Warrior 3 (left)

10 breaths x Sun God (see p. 63)

10 breaths x Standing Wide Leg Forward Bend

(see p. 67)

*Complete this circuit as many times as
you can in 20 minutes:*

5 x Yoga Push-ups (see p. 124)

10 x Star Jumps (see p. 139)

5 x Narrow Push-ups (see p. 123)

10 x Sumo Squats (see p. 136)

5 x Rocking Boats (see p. 154)

10 x Squat Jumps (see p. 138)

5 x Down Dog Push-ups (see p. 127)

10 x Mountain Climbers (see p. 145)

**1 ROUND**

30 breaths x Butterfly (see p. 167)

20 breaths each leg x Dragon (see p. 171)

20 breaths x Shoulder Stand (see p. 188)

**10 ROUNDS**

Square Breathing (see p. 56)

**1 ROUND**

15 breaths each side x Neck Release (see p. 178)

20 breaths x Ragdoll (see p. 164)

20 breaths x Toddler Squat (see p. 166)

20 breaths x Ragdoll

20 breaths x Straddle (see p. 169)

20 breaths x Butterfly (yin) (see p. 167)

20 breaths each leg x Shoelace (see p. 172)

20 breaths each leg x Deer (see p. 173)

20 breaths x Melting Heart (see p. 179)

20 breaths x Shoulder Stand (see p. 188)

10 breaths Plough (see p. 189)

100 breaths x Corpse (see p. 193)

## TIME TO TAKE STOCK

Now would be a good time to repeat the strength
and flexibility tests on page 12 to assess your
progress and make sure you're choosing the most
suitable variation of each pose and yogacise.
Share your progress using #YogaGym.

WEEK 3

**WEEK 3**

**SESSION 1**

**Focus:** Upper body

**Training type:** Tabatas

---

**3 ROUNDS**

Four Face Breathing (see p. 54)

---

# Warm-up C (see p. 200)

---

**3 ROUNDS**

5 breaths x Down Dog (see p. 80)

5 breaths x Plank (see p. 84)

5 breaths x Crocodile (see p. 88)

5 breaths x Up Dog (see p. 102)

5 breaths x Reverse Table Top (see p. 103)

---

**4 ROUNDS**

20 seconds x Half Down Dog Bombers (see p. 131)

*Push off a wall or elevate your hands on*

*a surface if you need to.*

Rest at 10 seconds

20 seconds x Bouncing Push-ups (see p. 126)

OR Classic Push-ups (see p. 122)

*Push off a wall or elevate your hands on*

*a surface if you need to.*

Rest at 10 seconds

20 seconds x Bear Crawl (see p. 133)

Rest at 10 seconds

20 seconds x Yoga Push-ups (see p. 124)

*Push off a wall or elevate your hands on*

*a surface if you need to.*

Rest at 10 seconds

20 seconds x Crab Walk (see p. 134)

Rest at 60 seconds

---

**1 ROUND**

Maximum number of Classic Push-ups in 1 minute

*Push off a wall or elevate your hands*

*on a surface if you need to.*

---

**1 ROUND**

10 breaths x Seagull Arms (see p. 190)

30 breaths x Melting Heart (see p. 179)

20 breaths each side x Thread The Needle (see p. 181)

10 breaths each side x Cow Face Arms (see p. 191)

**Focus:** Lower body

**Training type:** Tabatas

---

**1 ROUND**

10 breaths x Three Part Breath (see p. 55)

---

**Warm-up C** (see p. 200)

---

**1 ROUND**

10 breaths x Triangle (right) (see p. 68)

10 breaths x Side Angle (right) (see p. 70)

10 breaths x Warrior 2 (right) (see p. 73)

10 breaths x Warrior 1 (right) (see p. 72)

10 x Head to Knee (right) (see p. 66)

10 x Twisted Triangle (right) (see p. 69)

10 x Twisted Side Angle (right) (see p. 71)

Repeat all of the above on the left side.

---

**4 ROUNDS**

20 seconds x Reverse Lunge (see p. 141)

*4 each side then switch legs*

Rest @ 10 seconds

20 seconds x Squat Jumps (see p. 138)

Rest @ 10 seconds

20 seconds x Power Lunge (see p. 142)

*4 each side then switch legs*

Rest @ 10 seconds

20 seconds x Bear Crawl (see p. 133)

Rest @ 10 seconds

20 seconds x Pogo Jumps (see p. 149)

Rest @ 60 seconds

---

**1 ROUND**

Maximum number of Squats (see p. 135) in 1 minute

---

**1 ROUND**

20 breaths each side x Shoelace (see p. 172)

20 breaths each side x Sleeping Hero (see p. 174)

20 breaths each side x Sleeping Pigeon (see p. 170)

**Focus:** Core

**Training type:** Tabatas

**3 ROUNDS**

Stomach Pumping Breath (see p. 57)

# Warm-up D (see p. 200)

**1 ROUND**

10 breaths x Plank (see p. 84)

10 breaths x Low Boat (see p. 90)

10 breaths each side x Side Plank (see p. 85)

10 breaths x Locust (see p. 105)

10 breaths x Boat (see p. 89)

**4 ROUNDS**

20 seconds Flutter Kicks (see p. 160)

Rest @ 10 seconds

20 seconds Floating Straddle (see p. 161)

Rest @ 10 seconds

20 seconds Yogic Bicycles (see p.158)

Rest @ 10 seconds

20 seconds Iron Crosses (see p. 153)

Rest @ 10 seconds

20 seconds Locust Lifts (see p. 157)

Rest @ 60 seconds

**1 ROUND**

Maximum number of Crunches (see p. 159) in 1 minute

**1 ROUND**

20 breaths x Baby Cobra (yin) (see p. 183)

10 breaths each side x Sleeping Crocodile (see p. 184)

10 breaths x Camel (see p. 108)

20 breaths x Caterpillar (see p. 182)

15 breaths each side x Banana (see p. 184)

**1 ROUND**

2 minutes x Ocean Breath (see p. 53)

## Warm-up D (see p. 200)

**1 ROUND**

5 breaths x Bear (see p. 79)

10 breaths x Chair (see p. 62)

5 breaths each side x Twisted Chair (see p. 64)

10 breaths x Wide Leg Seated
Forward Bend (see p. 95)

5 breaths x Half Butterfly Forward Bend
(straight right leg) (see p. 96)

5 x Half Butterfly Side Bend (straight
right leg) (see p. 97)

5 breaths x Half Butterfly Twist
(straight right leg) (see p. 97)

5 breaths x Half Butterfly Forward Bend
(straight left leg) (see p. 97)

5 x Half Butterfly Side Bend (straight left leg) (see p. 97)

5 breaths x Half Butterfly Twist (straight
left leg) (see p. 97)

*Complete this circuit as many times as
you can in 20 minutes:*

10 x Half Down Dog Bombers (see p. 131)

10 x Squat Jumps (see p. 138)

10 x Flutter Kicks (see p. 160)

10 x Bear Bends (see p. 148)

10 x Yoga Push-ups (see p. 124)

10 x Mountain Climbers (see p. 145)

10 x Down Dog Push-ups (see p. 127)

10 x Star Jumps (see p. 139)

**1 ROUND**

20 breaths x Melting Heart (see p. 179)

20 breaths per leg x Dragon (see p. 171)

20 breaths x Butterfly (see p. 167)

20 breaths x Sleeping Butterfly (see p. 167)

20 breaths x Shoulder Stand (see p. 188)

**Focus:** Recovery

**Training type:** Yin

---

**10 ROUNDS**

Square Breathing (see p. 56)

---

**1 ROUND**

15 breaths each side x Neck Release (see p. 178)

15 breaths x Baby Cobra (yin) (see p. 183)

10 breaths x Sleeping Crocodile (right) (see p. 184)

15 breaths x Baby Cobra (yin)

10 breaths x Sleeping Crocodile (left)

20 breaths Child's Pose (see p. 180)

25 breaths x Sleeping Pigeon (right) (see p. 170)

25 breaths x Dragon (left) (see p. 171)

25 breaths x Sleeping Pigeon (left)

25 breaths x Dragon (right)

30 breaths x Butterfly (yin) (see p. 167)

10 breaths x Windshield Wipers (see p. 113)

20 breaths x Sleeping Hero (see p. 174)

10 breaths x Windshield Wipers (see p. 113)

10 breaths each side x Reclining Twist (see p. 186)

20 breaths x Shoulder Stand (see p. 188)

20 breaths x Plough (see p. 189)

100 breaths x Corpse (see p. 193)

**Focus:** Upper body

**Training type:** Intervals

---

**3 ROUNDS**

Four Face Breathing (see p. 54)

---

# Warm-up D (see p. 200)

---

**3 ROUNDS**

10 breaths x Plank (see p. 84)

5 breaths x Planche Plank (see p. 86)

5 breaths x Crow (see p. 87)

---

**3 ROUNDS**

10 x Yoga Push-up (see p. 124)

*Push off a wall or elevate your hands on a surface if you need to.*

Rest @ 60 seconds

---

**3 ROUNDS**

10 x Windmill Push-up (see p. 128)

*Push off a wall or elevate your hands on a surface if you need to.*

Rest @ 60 seconds

---

**3 ROUNDS**

10 x Down Dog Bomber (see p. 132)

*Push off a wall or elevate your hands on a surface if you need to.*

Rest @ 60 seconds

---

**3 ROUNDS**

10 x Bouncing Push-up (see p. 126) OR Classic Push-up (see p. 122)

*Push off a wall or elevate your hands on a surface if you need to.*

Rest @ 60 seconds

---

**1 ROUND**

Maximum number of Classic Push-ups in 1 minute

*Push off a wall or elevate your hands on a surface if you need to.*

---

**1 ROUND**

30 breaths x Melting Heart (see p. 179)

10 breaths x Reverse Prayer (see p. 192)

25 breaths each side x Thread The Needle (see p. 181)

---

WORK TO FAILURE IF YOU
CAN'T REACH 12 REPETITIONS
FOR EACH EXERCISE.

**WEEK 4**

**SESSION 2**

**Focus:** Lower body

**Training type:** Supersets

---

**1 ROUND**

10 rounds x Three Part Breath (see p. 55)

---

**Warm-up D** (see p. 200)

---

**1 ROUND**

10 breaths x Chair (see p. 62)

10 breaths x Sun God (see p. 63)

5 breaths Standing Forward Bend (see p. 65)

5 breaths x Seated Forward Bend (see p. 93)

5 breaths each leg x Screaming Pigeon (see p. 170)

5 breaths each leg x Screaming Dragon (see p. 99)

---

**3 ROUNDS**

6 x Squats (see p.135) with 3-second pause at the bottom

12 x Down Dog Jumps (see p. 150)

Rest @ 30 seconds

---

**3 ROUNDS**

6 x Sumo Squats (see p. 136) with

3-second pause at the bottom

12 x Star Jumps (see p. 139)

Rest @ 30 seconds

---

**3 ROUNDS**

6 each side x Split Squats (see p. 143)

with 3-second pause at the bottom

12 x Mountain Climbers (see p. 145)

Rest @ 30 seconds

---

**1 ROUND**

Maximum number of Squats (see p. 135) in 1 minute

---

**1 ROUND**

20 breaths each side x Dragon (see p. 171)

20 breaths each side x Sleeping Pigeon (see p. 170)

20 breaths x Straddle (see p. 169)

20 breaths x Butterfly (see p. 167)

**3 ROUNDS**

Stomach Pumping Breath (see p. 57)

**Warm-up D** (see p. 200)

**1 ROUND**

10 breaths x Plank (see p. 84)

10 breaths x Boat (see p. 89)

5 breaths x Crow (see p. 87)

10 breaths each side x Side Plank (see p. 85)

10 breaths x Baby Bridge (see p. 106)

5 breaths x Bridge (see p. 107)

**4 ROUNDS**

20 seconds x Iron Crosses (see p. 153)

Rest @ 10 seconds

20 seconds x Rocking Boats (see p. 154)

Rest @ 10 seconds

20 seconds x Flutter Kicks (see p. 160)

Rest @ 10 seconds

20 seconds x Floating Straddles (see p. 161)

Rest @ 10 seconds

20 seconds x Glute Bridges (see p. 147)

Rest @ 60 seconds

**1 ROUND**

Maximum number of Crunches (see p. 159) in 1 minute

**1 ROUND**

20 breaths x Up Dog (see p. 102)

10 breaths each side x Sleeping Crocodile (see p. 184)

20 breaths x Happy Baby (see p. 177)

10 breaths each side x Reclining Twist (see p. 186)

10 breaths each side x Banana (see p. 184)

**WEEK 4**

**SESSION 4**

**Focus:** Body blast

**Training type:** PHA training

---

**1 ROUND**

2 minutes x Ocean Breath (see p. 53)

---

# Warm-up D (see p. 200)

---

**1 ROUND**

10 breaths x Chair (see p. 62)

10 breaths each side x Eagle (see p. 77)

10 breaths x Standing Wide Leg Forward Bend (see p. 67)

10 breaths x Warrior 2 (right) (see p. 73)

10 breaths x Warrior 1 (right) (see p. 72)

10 breaths x Warrior 3 (right) (see p. 74)

10 breaths x Warrior 2 (left)

10 breaths x Warrior 1 (left)

10 breaths x Warrior 3 (left)

---

*Complete this circuit as many times as you can in 20 minutes:*

5 x Classic Push-ups (see p. 122)

10 x Squats (see p. 135)

5 x Down Dog Push-ups (see p. 127)

10 x Squat Jumps (see p. 138)

5 x Down Dog Bombers (see p. 132)

10 each leg x Lunges (see p. 140)

5 x Yoga Push-ups (see p. 124)

10 x Star Jumps (see p. 139)

---

**1 ROUND**

20 breaths x Ragdoll (see p. 164)

20 breaths x Toddler Squat (see p. 166)

20 breaths x Frog (see p. 175)

20 breaths x Shoulder Stand (see p. 188)

10 breaths x Plough (see p. 189)

---

**WEEK 4**

**SESSION 5**

**Focus:** Recovery

**Training type:** Yin

---

**10 ROUNDS**

Square Breathing (see p. 56)

---

**1 ROUND**

30 breaths x Butterfly (yin) (see p. 167)

20 breaths each leg x Half Butterfly (yin) (see p. 168)

30 breaths x Straddle (see p. 169)

10 breaths x Windshield Wipers (see p. 113)

20 breaths each side x Deer (see p. 173)

20 breaths x Baby Cobra (yin) (see p. 183)

20 breaths x Child's Pose (see p. 180)

20 breaths each side x Shoelace (see p. 172)

20 breaths each side x Sleeping Pigeon (see p. 170)

20 breaths each side x Eye of the Needle (see p. 176)

20 breaths each side x Reclining Twist (see p. 186)

30 breaths x Shoulder Stand (see p. 188)

100 breaths x Corpse (see p. 193)

---

## SEE HOW FAR YOU'VE COME!

Now would be a good time to repeat the strength and flexibility tests on page 12 and compare them to your test results before you started the plan to see you how far you have come. Share your progress with #YogaGym.

# Appendix

## Glossary

**Abdominal lock**   a gentle contraction of the abdomen above and below the belly button to stabilise the core and provide space for forward bends.

**Abdominals**   the large group of muscles between the chest and the pelvis that assist with breathing, posture and movement. Informally know as 'abs'.

**Agonist**   a muscle that contracts at the same time as another relaxes. For example, when bending the elbow, the bicep is the agonist.

**Antagonist**   a muscle that relaxes at the same time as another contracts. For example, when bending the elbow, the tricep is the antagonist.

**Biceps**   a large muscle at the front of the upper arm.

**Body composition**   the percentage of fat, muscle, bone and water in the body, which determines our leanness.

**Bottom position**   the point in an exercise where you have finished the eccentric part of the movement. For example, when squatting, the point where you have fully bent your knees and your bottom is as near as it can be to the ground.

**Calisthenics**   exercises that are done in a systematic way using the bodyweight for resistance.

**Calf**   the muscle between the knee and ankle on the back of the lower leg.

**Cartilage**   a tough and flexible connective tissue found in various parts of the body including the surfaces of joints.

**Co-contract**   simultaneously contracting two or more muscles to stabilise a joint and provide stillness in a pose

**Collagen**   the main component of connective tissues such as ligaments, tendons and fascia, which gives these tissues their tensile strength.

**Compound movement**   movements or exercises that use more than one joint or muscle group at a time. For example, a squat uses quadriceps, hamstrings, abdominals, gluteals and lower back muscles.

**Concentric muscle contraction**   a type of muscle contraction in which the muscles shorten at the same time as generating force. For example, bending your elbow requires concentric contraction of the biceps.

**Core**   every muscle in your body apart from your arms and legs, including your abdominals, pelvic floor, obliques, diaphragm and back muscles.

**Counter pose**   a pose that moves the body in the opposite direction from the one it was in during the previous pose, to return the spine to a neutral position.

**Diaphragm**   the sheet of muscle between the abdomen and chest that is responsible for breathing.

**Eccentric muscle contraction**   a type of muscle contraction in which the muscles lengthen at the same time as generating force. For example, straightening the arm with control requires eccentric contraction of the bicep.

**Edge**   the point in a yoga pose just outside your comfort zone where you are working with enough intensity and challenge to create strength and flexibility without straining or feeling pain.

**Elliptical trainer**   a stationary exercise machine used to simulate stair climbing or walking. Also known as a cross-trainer.

**Erector spinae**   a group of muscles running parallel to the spinal column that extend the spine and provide resistance that assists the control of a bending-forwards motion at the waist.

**Extension**   a straightening movement that increases the angle between body parts. For example, standing up from a forward bend is an extension of the spine.

**Fibroblast**   the most common cells of connective tissues, which produce collagen and other fibres.

**Flexion**   a bending movement that decreases the angle between body parts. For example, folding forwards to touch your toes requires flexion of the spine.

**Gluteal muscles**   a group of muscles that make up the buttocks, including the gluteus maximus, gluteus medius, gluteus minimus and tensor fasciae latae.

**Hamstrings**   a group of muscles located at the back of the thigh that are responsible for knee flexion and hip extension.

**Heart centre**   the centre of the chest. This is often used as a cue in poses such as backbends to encourage the lifting of the chest forwards to achieve an even curve throughout the spine.

**Hip flexors**   a group of muscles at the front of the hip, including the psoas, iliacus and rectus femoris, that bring the legs and hips together in a flexion movement.

**Homeostasis**   the maintenance of a constant internal environment in the body, including temperature control and water balance.

**Hyperextension**   the extension of a body part beyond its normal limits to increase strength and flexibility.

**Hypertrophy**   an increase in the size of a muscle.

**Inversion**   a type of yoga pose in which the head is below the heart. For example, Headstand, Handstand and Shoulder Stand.

**Interval training**   a form of high intensity training which involves short periods of intense exercise followed by short periods of rest.

**Isometric muscle contraction**   a type of muscle contraction in which there is no movement at a joint and the muscle does not change in length. For example, pushing against a wall.

**Lateral flexion or motion**   movement of the spine in a sideways motion. For example, bending sideways at the waist.

**Macronutrient**   nutrients that provide calories for energy, growth, and bodily functions. There are three macronutrients: protein, carbohydrate, and fat.

**Oblique muscles**   muscles on either side of the torso that assist with side-bending and rotation.

**Osteoblast**   a cell that makes bone.

**Pelvic floor**   a muscular partition at the base of the abdomen thart provides support for the bladder, intestines, and uterus (in women).

**Periodisation**   the organisation of training into blocks that focus on different goals.

**Peripheral Heart Action (PHA) Training**   a form of training designed to keep blood circulating throughout the body by performing an upper body exercise followed by a lower body exercise.

**Perpendicular**   at a right angle to a given surface or to the ground.

**Plyometric**   a movement or exercise in which the muscles are stretched and then contracted to improve power. For example, jumping high off the ground.

**Posterior kinetic chain**   a series of muscles in the back of the body, including the lower back muscles, gluteal muscles, hamstrings and calves.

**Progressive overload**   the gradual increase in stress placed on the body during a training plan to stimulate increases in muscle size, strength, endurance, flexibility and overall fitness.

**Quadriceps**   the muscles at the front of the thigh that extend the knee and flex the hip. Also known as 'quads'.

**Repetitions**   the number of times to perform an exercise before stopping or moving on to the next exercise. Also known as 'reps'.

**Sets**   the numbers of times to perform the exercise for the number of repetitions. For example three sets of 12 repetitions.

**S-curve**   the natural curve of the spine, which resembles a soft 'S' shape when viewed from the side.

**Stretch reflex**   a muscle contraction that attempts to resist the change in muscle length caused by stretching.

**Supersets**   two exercises performed back to back without any rest.

**Synergistic**   working together. Treating the body as one unit rather than dividing it into individual muscle groups.

**Synovial fluid**   a lubricating fluid found in synovial joints, such as the shoulder, knee and hip.

**Tabata**   a form of high intensity interval training involving exercising for 20 seconds and resting for 10 seconds.

**Triceps**   the large muscle at the back of the upper arm.

**Top position**   the position in which you start and finish an exercise.

**Yogacise**   a yoga-based bodyweight exercise used to achieve bodily fitness and grace of movement.

# Index

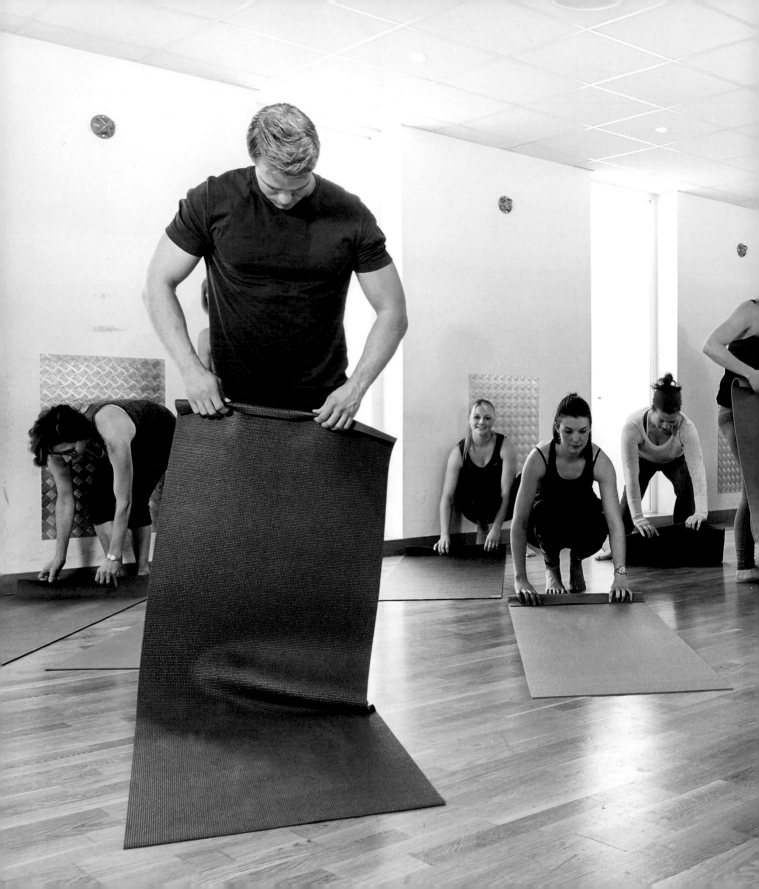

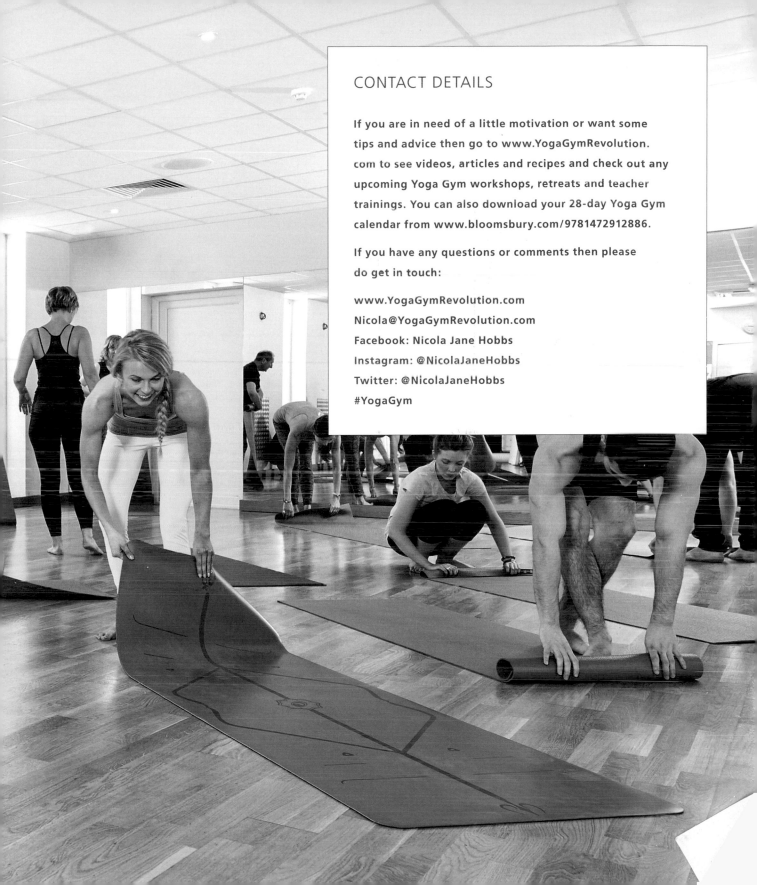

## CONTACT DETAILS

If you are in need of a little motivation or want some tips and advice then go to www.YogaGymRevolution. com to see videos, articles and recipes and check out any upcoming Yoga Gym workshops, retreats and teacher trainings. You can also download your 28-day Yoga Gym calendar from www.bloomsbury.com/9781472912886.

If you have any questions or comments then please do get in touch:

www.YogaGymRevolution.com
Nicola@YogaGymRevolution.com
Facebook: Nicola Jane Hobbs
Instagram: @NicolaJaneHobbs
Twitter: @NicolaJaneHobbs
#YogaGym